PAIN KILLER

PAIN
KILLER

A "Wonder" Drug's
Trail of Addiction
and Death

BARRY
MEIER

RODALE

© 2003 by Barry Meier

Printed in the United States of America
Rodale Inc. makes every effort to use acid-free ∞, recycled paper ♻.

Book design by Christopher Rhoads

Library of Congress Cataloging-in-Publication Data

Meier, Barry.
  Pain killer : a "wonder" drug's trail of addiction and death / Barry Meier.
     p. ; cm.
  ISBN 1–57954–638–2 hardcover
  1. Oxycodone—United States.   2. Medication abuse—United States.
I. Title.
  [DNLM: 1. Oxycodone—poisoning.   2. Drug Industry—standards.
3. Opioid-Related Disorders—epidemiology.   4. Opioid-Related
Disorders—mortality.   5. Oxycodone—history.   6. Street Drugs—
supply & distribution.
QV 92 M511p   2003]
HV5822.O99M45   2003
362.29'9—dc22   2003015003

Distributed to the book trade by St. Martin's Press
2   4   6   8   10   9   7   5   3   1   hardcover

Visit us on the Web at www.rodalestore.com, or call us toll-free at (800) 848-4735.

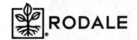

WE **INSPIRE** AND **ENABLE** PEOPLE TO IMPROVE
THEIR LIVES AND THE WORLD AROUND THEM

For Ellen and Lily

ACKNOWLEDGMENTS

Every book requires a leap of faith on the part of a large number of people. This book was no different. A remarkable number of people willingly gave of their time, talents, insights, energy, enthusiasm, and helpful criticism.

Jane Dystel, my agent, worked hard, and Stephanie Tade, my editor at Rodale, took a gamble. Susan Leon guided my writing and Barbara Mantel did valuable research. Chris Potash had sound editing suggestions, and Anne Hurley, Adam Liptak, and David McCraw looked at an early manuscript with fresh eyes.

Walt Bogdanich, my colleague and friend at the *New York Times*, first mentioned OxyContin to me, setting me on this path. Melody Petersen and I worked together and the *Times* allowed me to draw from our reporting. The paper's management and Glenn Kramon, the business editor, gave me the gift of time.

The Kaiser Family Foundation awarded me a generous fellowship. Penny Duckham of Kaiser is a journalist's ally extraordinaire. I hope that Penny, Hale Champion, Paul Delaney, Dr. Timothy Johnson, and Bill Kovach will see this book as a repayment for their leap of faith.

Many other people took another kind of leap. They opened

their lives or shared their knowledge. There are far too many to mention by name, but Art Van Zee, Sue Ella Kobak, Jane Myers, Lindsay Myers, Russell Portenoy, Sister Beth Davies, Larry Lavender, and Laura Nagel deserve special thanks. Also, Nathaniel Paul Katz spent hours helping me better understand pain treatment, and Gregory Wood's daily news roundups were invaluable. A number of former Purdue officials shared their experiences. I'm grateful for their leap of faith.

My family and friends aided and abetted me in countless ways. Jill Abramson and Henry Griggs were great hosts, and Harriet Grimm and Elissa Krauss constantly opened their home to my daughter, Lily, so that she and Sylvia could play. A special note of thanks to my brother, Steve, my sister-in-law, Iris Osman, my mother, Gerta, and my mother-in-law, Iris Pollock.

In the end, there is one person who made this all possible: my wife, Ellen. She kept me together from the start to the end, and at every step along the way. My debt is such that neither chocolate nor jewelry can ever repay it. Nonetheless, I'll try.

Finishing a book provides a great sense of satisfaction. Getting back to Ellen and Lily offers a bigger one. I've missed you both more than you can imagine.

CONTENTS

PAIN KILLER

THE BOOK OF THE DEAD

DR. FREDRIC HELLMAN had long kept his own book of the dead. Slightly oversized and covered in blue cloth, it was the type of ledger that a book-keeper might use to tabulate and balance accounts. In it, the medical examiner recorded every unexplained, mysterious, or violent death he worked on. He had small, meticulous handwriting, and every case entered into the book was accorded its own line. Running down the columns were identification numbers, dates, ages, sexes, autopsy findings, laboratory test results, and, finally, the cause of death.

Hellman liked having all this data in one book because it helped him spot patterns. Toward the end of 2000 he noticed a new one emerging from death's steady background noise. In the small county south of Philadelphia where Hellman worked, a drug called oxycodone was turning up in the blood and urine of overdose victims. The oddly named chemical was actually legal. It was a painkilling narcotic long used as the active ingredient in a variety of prescription medications sold under names such as Percocet, Percodan, and Tylox.

Hellman wasn't a stranger to the drug. He typically performed about five hundred autopsies each year, and oxycodone would turn up in two or three. This year, though, was different. In just one month it had been found during four autopsies. By the time Hellman closed his ledger on 2000, the painkiller had been detected in connection with fifteen deaths, sometimes at toxic dosages, more frequently in combination with alcohol and other prescription drugs.

A state medical examiner in Roanoke, Virginia, some 360 miles to the south, was seeing the same thing. Dr. William Massello's encounters with oxycodone, much like Hellman's, had once been limited. But in 1999, the painkiller had figured in eleven autopsies. From there, the numbers had shot up like the line on a fever chart: the body count rose to sixteen in 2000 and to forty in 2001.

It wasn't just the death toll that was mounting. Linda Sullivan noticed that the faces of the dead were changing. Sullivan helped run a testing lab that did work for medical examiners throughout Florida. She had long associated high oxycodone levels at death with older patients who had been given the drug to help ease their suffering from painful diseases such as cancer. But during the summer of 2000, many of those dying in Florida with the drug in their system were in their early twenties, an age group not generally associated with terminal illness or severe pain.

Sullivan called medical examiners to ask a series of probing questions. Had investigators found prescriptions for painkillers containing oxycodone at the death scenes? Were doctors treating the overdose victims for pain? Time after time she got the same response: no.

Soon others started asking similar questions. Over time their ranks would grow to include drug company executives, physicians, pharmacists, lawmakers, pain patients, cops, drug abusers, and kids just looking for a thrill. Together they formed an army of unknowing volunteers, each playing his or her part in a massive and unplanned public health experiment. It was an experiment that involved one of the most potentially addicting narcotics ever legally sold. Its brand name was OxyContin.

At its birth, OxyContin had been a pharmaceutical industry dream, a "wonder" that heralded a sea change in the treatment of pain. For more than a decade, a determined band of medical specialists had carefully laid the groundwork for the painkiller's appearance by waging a campaign to draw attention to pain— mankind's oldest and most persistent medical enemy. Outdated fears about the potential of narcotics to cause abuse, these pain warriors declared, were causing millions of patients to suffer unnecessarily. OxyContin was the answer to their pleas; it promised not only a better approach to pain relief, but a safer one as well. Soon, the drug's producer made the painkiller the centerpiece of the biggest and most aggressive marketing campaign for a powerful narcotic in modern pharmaceutical history. Within just a few years of its launch in 1996, OxyContin was a blockbuster, with annual sales of more than a billion dollars.

For a time it must have appeared that all the right stars had come into alignment. The fight against pain had intensified and was seemingly being won. Vast profits and careers were being made. But the era of OxyContin also set into motion forces that were far from celestial. In fact, they had already gathered to form a perfect medical storm.

CHAPTER ONE

PILL HILL

LATE ON A JANUARY night in 2000, the telephone rang in the bedroom of a country doctor named Art Van Zee. He picked it up quickly and listened while a nurse at a nearby hospital explained that a young woman had just been brought into the emergency room after overdosing on a painkiller. She was now in the intensive care unit on a respirator.

It was Van Zee's night on call, so he eased out of bed, quietly dressed, and left the house. Slowly he drove his car down a long, twisting dirt driveway, past the man-made trout pond and the corral that was home to his children's ponies and donkeys. At the end of the road he passed the small concrete building that served as his wife's law office, then turned right onto a two-lane highway that led from Dryden, Virginia, where he lived, to Pennington Gap, a town of eighteen hundred where Lee County Community Hospital was located.

At the time, Art Van Zee was fifty-two. He had grown up thousands of miles away from this slice of Appalachia, in the small, high-desert city of Elko, Nevada. But after twenty-five years of living in Lee County he had come to love everything about the region—its landscape, its culture, and its separateness. Over time he had become part of this place, and it in turn had embraced him.

Lee County lies in southwestern Virginia, wedged between Kentucky and Tennessee, deep in coal country. It is a place of breathtaking beauty as well as intense poverty. The Cumberland Mountains run through its heart and, over time, fast-running streams have sliced deeply through them, forming a landscape of steep, stony mountain ridges, plunging hollows, and gentle valleys. Stands of loblolly pine, shortleaf pine, hickory, and oak rise out of the soil. Below the land are thick, rich veins of coal, a source of Appalachia's wealth and also much of its heartache. Just over the Kentucky border from Lee County, for example, is Harlan County, the scene of several violent and bloody mineworker strikes, including one in 1974 that became the subject of the Oscar-winning documentary *Harlan County USA*.

Art Van Zee had first come to Lee County that same year as part of a contingent of Vanderbilt University medical students that traveled throughout Appalachia giving free physical examinations to people who rarely got them. Two years later he came back, this time as a volunteer in a government program that sends doctors into poor areas that have few physicians. Van Zee started running a community heath clinic in the small town of St. Charles, Virginia, which lies at the intersection of several small roads and railroad spurs.

As recently as the 1950s, St. Charles had been an Appalachian boomtown, its streets lined with a hotel, a bank, movie theaters, and restaurants. But by the time Van Zee arrived, in 1976, coal-digging machines had displaced many miners and St. Charles was already fast on its way to becoming a ghost town of shuttered stores.

Mining was still a part of the region, though. Scores of families continued to live in the hardscrabble coal camps—collections of shacks, tar-paper shanties, and broken-down homes that line the roads leading to the mine gates. Ear-piercing squeals often screamed through those camps like errant pieces of blackboard chalk, sounds caused by the slow, grinding iron wheels of railway boxcars as long lines of the containers were eased under hoppers so they could be loaded with coal.

Wayne A. Van Zee, who was known to everyone as Art, could have chosen to practice anywhere. But his father was a Presbyterian minister who had instilled in him the notion that work should be a form of service. And so Wayne A. Van Zee, a tall, gangly man with a salt-and-pepper beard, performed his job in Lee County with a missionary's intensity.

Ever since he had arrived, Van Zee had tried to do whatever he could to improve health care in an area where medical services are painfully scarce. He had organized smoking cessation contests. He had brought in experts to perform cancer screenings and to give mammograms. He had run fairs that offered prenatal care. He had even put together courses on healthier cooking, a hard sell in a part of the country where anything edible runs the risk of being fried. Each year, thousands of people passed through the St. Charles clinic to get treated for every imaginable illness. For those too sick to come in, Van Zee made house calls, driving out to the coal camps. When mining disasters struck, he'd stand duty at the mouth of the pits even when the only help he could give was to those who were recovering bodies. His was an all-consuming job. According to one local story, Van Zee's car was found blocking traffic in town one night, with him asleep inside. He had passed out from exhaustion while waiting for a red light to change. Fortunately, on this January night, he had rested.

It took Van Zee about fifteen minutes to reach Lee County Hospital, a small but modern-looking facility. The young woman, he was told, had overdosed on a narcotic painkiller called OxyContin. She had been visiting her parents when she had fallen out of bed with such a thump that they had raced into her room. They found her lying on the floor, comatose and close to death. Narcotic painkillers depress the respiratory system, and most fatalities involving such drugs occur because people stop breathing. To save the woman's life, hospital physicians had put an emergency breathing tube down her throat and connected it to a respirator.

Van Zee had little firsthand experience with OxyContin, a timed-release painkiller similar in strength to morphine. The medication was still relatively new to the marketplace, and he had prescribed it only a few times, typically to patients suffering from cancer or those who had undergone numerous surgeries for constant, searing back pain without finding relief. Van Zee knew just about everybody in Lee County, so he glanced at the young woman lying asleep under the bedsheet to see if he recognized her. At first he didn't because the respirator mask obscured her face. He picked up her chart and then it hit him. Her name. Twenty-one years before, he had first held her as a three-month-old baby and had given her immunization shots. Over the years he had treated her for childhood illnesses and had watched her grow into a teenager who had thrived in high school.

He took a deep breath and blew it out. Van Zee had been told by a local drug abuse counselor and an area druggist in recent months that they were getting worried because OxyContin had started showing up for sale on the street. Van Zee hadn't paid much attention to their concerns; he'd always been very conservative when it came to prescribing drugs. He also had an extraordinary level of faith in the medical profession. It never would have occurred to him, for example, that not all doctors were so scrupulous. People who worked with Van Zee cherished his trusting nature, although they also suspected that the same quality caused him at times to be naïve.

Now, he looked down at the girl. He had known her all her life, and until this moment the last thing he would have ever expected to treat her for was a narcotic overdose. It was right about then that Art Van Zee began to wonder whether he needed to start worrying about OxyContin too.

It had taken grown-ups like Art Van Zee a long time to even begin to suspect what teenagers had known for nearly a year—that a tablet of OxyContin, or an Oxy, as they called it, was the ticket to a great high.

Another teenager was Lindsay Myers. Lindsay couldn't claim to be User Zero. But back in the spring of 1999, she took a certain pride in being among the youngest Oxy users she knew.

At the time, Lindsay was a sixteen-year-old sophomore at Lee County High School. She was a cheerleader for Lee High's football team, the Generals, and also ran track. Lindsay had a round, pretty face and her brown eyes were offset by dark blond hair, which she pulled back into a ponytail. She was the kind of girl boys noticed. Fate had treated her kindly in other respects as well. She came from one of the wealthiest families around. Her mother's father had founded a company that operated coal mines in Kentucky and Virginia and Lindsay's father, Johnny, had followed him into the mining business. While most kids at Lee High walked to school or were lucky to drive hand-me-downs, she tooled around in a brand-new black Jeep Cherokee. It was a far better car than her teachers could afford.

Lindsay lived in a large, modern house overlooking the town of Pennington Gap, a home that looked more like an upper-class dwelling in suburban Atlanta than small-town Appalachia. She wished it had been in Atlanta, a seven-hour drive to the south. Lindsay loved visiting the city on shopping trips with her mother, Jane, or, better yet, to attend rock concerts there with friends. Like most teenagers in Pennington Gap, she felt bored. There wasn't much to do, see, or buy. Its tiny downtown, really just two blocks straddling railroad tracks, had only a few stores. One of them, Gibson's, displayed flowered dresses of a style last seen decades earlier in big cities.

For teenagers like Lindsay, most of the action took place at the east end of town, where a two-lane road entered Pennington Gap. Fast-food restaurants stood clustered near the intersection. Kids from Lee High liked to hang out at McDonald's, while Hardee's attracted a slightly older crowd. Before long, Lindsay started hanging out there too.

Lindsay liked being around older kids, particularly those in their early or mid-twenties. They threw better parties and made her feel more grown up. They also had drugs, or knew where to get them.

She had tried her first Oxy while riding around in a car outside Pennington Gap. Lindsay watched as her friend popped a small blue tablet into his mouth and let it sit there for a few minutes before taking it out and wiping it off on his T-shirt. He then dropped the pill onto a creased dollar bill and folded the bill so that it formed a tight, tiny envelope, which he shoved back into his mouth. Next, he bit down on the package with his back teeth. Finally, the boy unfolded the bill and dumped the powdered contents onto a plastic compact disc holder so that he, Lindsay, and another friend could snort it.

Lindsay didn't get high that first time, though that didn't stop her. Friends kept raving about OxyContin, and soon one told her about someone dealing Oxys in Harlan, Kentucky, which was just a thirty-minute drive from Pennington Gap. The two took off in Lindsay's Jeep and soon found the address they were looking for, stopping the car in front of a darkened house. Lindsay handed the girl $150 and waited until her friend came back with four pills. On the drive home, the girls pulled off the road, crushed up the pills, and snorted them. Lindsay first felt sick to her stomach. But the nausea quickly passed and a rush of warmth spread through her body as all her muscles relaxed. Every tension, every care evaporated. She loved it; nothing she had ever tried before had made her feel that way. Back in Pennington Gap, the two girls cruised the main drag for a while. Then Lindsay started feeling sleepy. By the time she got home she couldn't keep her eyes open. She was getting still higher as a delicious cocoon of sleep wrapped around her.

The recreational use of prescription narcotics was nothing new in Lee County, or in many other parts of the country for that matter. But there was something new and very different about OxyContin. Its active ingredient—oxycodone—is the same narcotic found in some traditional painkillers such as Percodan, Percocet, and Tylox. But while those drugs typically contained 5 milligrams of oxycodone, the weakest version of OxyContin contained twice that amount. From there, the amount of oxycodone in different dosage strengths of OxyContin rose exponentially, to 20, 40, 80, and 160 milligrams. In terms of narcotic firepower, OxyContin was a nuclear weapon.

OxyContin was first sold in 1996 by a little-known Connecticut drugmaker named Purdue Frederick, which five years earlier had created a special unit called Purdue Pharma to market it. To create OxyContin, Purdue used a patented timed-release formula to pack large amounts of oxycodone into the drug. The round tablets released part of a pill's narcotic payload within the first hour and the rest over the next eleven hours. That gave OxyContin an edge over traditional narcotics, whose painkilling effect, while felt more quickly, lasted only around four hours. Most significantly, OxyContin delivered steadier and longer relief, granting patients in great pain the godsend of a regular night's sleep.

But Purdue also claimed that OxyContin's time-release mechanism would likely make it less appealing to those who abused painkillers. The company thinking was that to drug abusers the attractiveness of any particular substance is largely based on two factors: its strength and the speed with which it produces its effect. Given that OxyContin slowly released its oxycodone, officials of both Purdue and the Food and Drug Administration, the federal agency that must approve a prescription drug for sale, had thought that anyone seeking the euphoric rush of a narcotic would continue to favor traditional immediate-release painkillers. The trouble was that it didn't take long for even novice drug abusers like Lindsay Myers to discover that once an OxyContin tablet had been softened up with a little water or saliva, a good set of teeth could be used to crush the tablet, releasing its oversized narcotic trove for their immediate pleasure.

About a month after Lindsay had first tried an Oxy, she was

scoring one or two almost every day. She bought most of them from a woman nicknamed "Shorty" who lived in a small dilapidated house near the center of Pennington Gap. No one knew where Shorty got her drug, but it certainly wasn't through legitimate channels. OxyContin, because it contained oxycodone, fell within the category of the most powerful and potentially addictive painkillers legally available; they were also the most tightly controlled. Under federal law, every gram of these substances—formally known as Schedule II narcotics—manufactured, shipped, stocked in pharmacies, or prescribed by a doctor had to be logged in and accounted for. OxyContin's classmates in Schedule II included all the heaviest hitters: morphine, Dilaudid, and fentanyl.

For a long time, Lindsay never went inside Shorty's house. She just waited in her Jeep until the short, dark-haired woman came out. Then she handed Shorty cash and got her Oxys. Sometimes when there were too many cars outside her house, Shorty, to avoid attracting attention, would chase Lindsay and everyone away. Then one day in the summer of 1999 she invited Lindsay inside. Lindsay had expected the house to be trashy, like the way she imagined a dealer's den, but it had a warm, cozy feeling. She got to like Shorty, and pretty soon they started having coffee together and chatting. Before very long, Lindsay came to feel more relaxed at Shorty's than she did at her own home.

That summer, Lindsay just hung out and got high. She'd pick up friends and drive out of Pennington Gap on a narrow country lane called Skaggs Hill Road that meandered through rugged farm country before circling back to town. Skaggs Hill was known as Pill Hill. Lindsay and her friends would pull off on one of the road's many turnouts, crush up some Oxys, and snort them. The word about Oxys was spreading quickly; there would be times when Lindsay saw a different car pulled alongside Skaggs Hill Road every quarter mile or so.

It was during the Fourth of July weekend that Lindsay got her first glimpse of the drug's dark side. Every year her uncle hosted a family reunion at his lakefront summer home in Tennessee. Lindsay hadn't taken any Oxys along, and that first night at her uncle's house her legs began to hurt badly. Even as she lay in bed, she couldn't keep them from shaking.

"Mom, my legs are hurting so bad!" Lindsay called out. "Would you rub on them?"

Jane, her mother, came into Lindsay's room and started massaging her daughter's legs. The next night the pain was worse, so Jane went to a local drugstore and asked the pharmacist about Lindsay's symptoms. He thought she might be having leg cramps and recommended an over-the-counter medicine.

Lindsay's cramps weren't cured until she got back to Pennington Gap. She drove over to Shorty's house, bought an Oxy, and did it. That night she did two more and went to sleep. She awoke the next morning feeling good—and a little scared. She hadn't thought she could become addicted to the pills, at least not this easily. Later that day Lindsay told Shorty that she might be hooked.

Jane Myers didn't know anything about Shorty. But by the fall of 1999 she had started to worry about her daughter, who had been so beautiful and so energetic. Nowadays, Lindsay was having trouble getting up in the morning. Her interest in school had also fallen off, and she had quit the track team. When Jane had asked Lindsay why, she said she just didn't feel like doing it anymore.

During the summer, Jane's sister, who lived nearby, had told her that she had seen Lindsay hanging out with an older girl who had a reputation for doing drugs. She suggested that Jane find Lindsay a summer job, maybe one at the office of the family's coal business.

Jane, a reserved and attractive woman with red hair, hadn't paid her sister much mind. The idea of Lindsay doing drugs was inconceivable to her. Sure, she was a teenager and maybe going through some kind of phase, but Jane believed that she and her husband had done everything to make Lindsay happy. Like any parent of a teenager, she didn't want to intrude too much on Lindsay's privacy; Jane thought her daughter was at an age where she deserved more independence. If there was a real problem, she honestly believed that Lindsay would talk to her about it.

Besides, Lindsay hadn't given up cheerleading and seemed to enjoy it as much as ever. And Jane loved to watch her daughter perform; she'd often drive her to away games even if it sometimes meant a three-hour trip each way. One day that fall, it was already evening when Jane and Lindsay got home from a game. Lindsay's brother, Brandon, who was five years older, was hanging out with some of his friends in the basement, listening to music. As soon as Lindsay walked in the door, she threw her bag onto the kitchen table and went down to join them.

Jane looked at Lindsay's bag and decided on impulse to open it. Inside she found a small tablet and a thin metal tube about an inch long. Jane didn't have a clue what either of them was.

"Lindsay," she called downstairs, "I want to ask you something."

Lindsay came up and looked nonchalantly at the pill that her mother held.

"Oh, I haven't been able to sleep," she said. "Kimberly gave me that to help."

With that, she went back downstairs. Kimberly, Lindsay's cousin, was also at the house that night.

"Did you give Lindsay this?" she asked the girl.

"I haven't given her anything," Kimberly replied.

Jane felt her stomach drop. She shouted for Lindsay to come back up.

"Kim didn't give you this pill," she said. "What is it?"

"It's an Oxy," Lindsay said, with an obstinate, almost challenging look.

"And what's this?" said Jane, holding up the short, hollow tube.

"That's what I use to snort it," said Lindsay.

Jane panicked. Lindsay stormed off into her room and Jane told her to stay there. The next morning Jane called Beth Davies, who ran the local substance abuse clinic in Pennington Gap. Davies said she didn't know much about OxyContin, but she told Jane that the only way to really know what was going on was to have Lindsay's urine screened. Jane balked at the idea. She told Beth that making Lindsay submit to such a test wasn't fair; if someone found out she had been tested, she'd be followed around by rumors. Her school record might be blemished. She might even be thrown off the cheerleading squad. No, she just couldn't do that. By the end of their conversation Jane had agreed, however, to bring Lindsay in on Monday to Davies' office for a talk.

Beth Davies was about as unlikely a substance abuse counselor as one might find. In 1999 she was sixty-six years old but she looked a good decade younger and had the energy of someone half her age. A small, feisty woman with a gravelly voice and a shock of short silver hair, she was also a nun. Sister Beth, as many people called her, had first come to Appalachia in 1972 after spending a career as a teacher and administrator of parochial schools in New York and Connecticut. She arrived in St. Charles and helped lead the fund-raising drive to build the clinic where Art Van Zee now worked. A social activist, she also became involved in environmental battles and other issues.

Then, in 1979, Davies lost her own long-running battle with alcoholism. She entered a church-owned treatment facility in Massachusetts for nuns with substance abuse problems and decided again to change careers. She first went to Rutgers University in New Jersey for training, then spent a year in Trenton's roughest neighborhoods counseling alcoholics and heroin addicts.

Ever since the mid-1980s, Beth and Elizabeth Vines, another nun who had battled alcoholism, had run the Addiction Education Center in an old two-story building in downtown Pennington Gap. Initially the two worked almost exclusively with alcoholics, but by the early 1990s they were seeing an increase in the abuse of prescription medications such as tranquilizers, like Valium and Xanax, and painkillers. Those drugs included not only Percocet and Tylox but other pain medications sold under brand names like Vicodin and Lortab that contained a narcotic called hydrocodone. Compounds like Vicodin were prescribed far more widely than drugs like Percocet that used oxycodone because hydrocodone was perceived to pose a lower addiction risk than oxycodone and federal regulations governing its prescription were less stringent. By the fall of 1999 both Beth and Elizabeth had also begun to hear about Oxy-Contin from a few people seeking help. But nothing could have prepared them for what they were about to face.

For Lindsay, the weekend wait before her appointment with Davies was agonizing; she was going through the brutal experience known as withdrawal. People who take a narcotic for a while develop a physical dependence on it, and their bodies will go into some degree of shock if that supply is suddenly cut off. Withdrawal is especially traumatic when high dosages are involved, and for Lindsay, who had been doing three Oxys a day—one before school, one at lunch, and one before cheerleading practice—it was excruciating. Her legs ached and jerked far more painfully than they had at her uncle's. Like a severe case of the flu, she trembled with chills, her nose and eyes ran, and she suffered blinding headaches. She even suffered through periods of delirium. One night that weekend Lindsay dreamed she had found an Oxy in her room and snorted it. When she woke up and realized it hadn't happened, she began to cry.

By the time Monday rolled around, Lindsay was looking forward to seeing Beth. Her mother hadn't really told her much about the drug counselor, but Lindsay assumed that Beth was young because her name sounded that way. Lindsay even imagined that Beth might be like a slightly older friend, someone with whom she could talk. So Lindsay sat quietly in Jane's Mercedes as the pair drove downtown. But as soon as Lindsay walked into Beth's office and saw her, she shut down. There was no way they could ever connect, she decided. Beth was too old.

"Can you tell me why you are here?" Beth had asked.

"I haven't done anything," Lindsay said.

"Apparently something is concerning your mother or she wouldn't have called," Beth replied. "What do you think it is?"

"I'm okay," Lindsay said. "She's really making too much of this. She wanted me to come, so that's why I'm here."

Lindsay and Beth never developed a bond. But for a month, at least, Lindsay managed to stay clean. Then one afternoon she was cruising around town and saw a girlfriend at a gas station. Lindsay pulled in and the girl gave her a big hug.

"Man, I wish I could find something," Lindsay said.

"You're in luck," her friend replied.

Years later, no one around Lee County would be able to pinpoint the precise moment in 2000 when they realized that an epidemic of OxyContin abuse had exploded in their midst. Not physicians like Art Van Zee. Not drug counselors like Beth Davies. Not law enforcement officials. But suddenly, as the winter of that year slid into spring, Oxys seemed to be everywhere.

Six months earlier, the drug had accounted for just a small fraction of the undercover drug buys by police officials in southwestern Virginia, but by April that figure had skyrocketed in some areas to 90 percent. It seemed to be coming from a variety of sources: a few unscrupulous doctors were selling prescriptions, other doctors were getting fooled by drug abusers feigning pain, and prescriptions for the painkiller were being forged, copied, or stolen.

For both habitual drug abusers and recreational users, OxyContin's purity was another reason it was so attractive. Traditional oxycodone-containing painkillers like Percodan or Tylox contained a combination of the narcotic and an over-the-counter analgesic, aspirin in the case of Percodan and acetaminophen in the case of both Tylox and Percocet. But OxyContin was pure oxycodone. That allowed pain patients to take large quantities of it without concerns of developing liver damage, a risk of both aspirin and acetaminophen. But the drug's purity also permitted both recreational users and drug abusers to easily snort it like cocaine or inject it like heroin. On the black market OxyContin had a value of $1 per milligram, meaning that a 20-milligram-strength tablet sold for $20 and a 40-milligram tablet sold for $40. Soon the demand for traditional painkillers seemed to dry up in Lee County and other places. It was as though some exotic new specimen had quietly slipped into the stream of drug abuse and driven out the native species.

For a few people like Lindsay Myers, finding the cash to buy Oxys wasn't a problem; she had thousands of dollars in her bank account when she first started using the drug. But most people didn't have that kind of money, and as OxyContin abuse accelerated, so did crime. Homes were broken into. Cash and televisions were stolen. In some cases, cancer and pain patients awoke to find bottles of OxyContin missing from their medicine cabinets. Forged, stolen, and worthless checks began to paper the region. So many of them were for $40—the street price of an Oxy 40—that area cops would joke upon finding one, "We know where that $40 went." People eager to get the drug ran up huge debts on their credit cards, buying things they could quickly convert into cash. Those without credit lines simply shoplifted items like cigarette lighters or compact discs from convenience stores or the local Wal-Mart and sold them for cash. In rural southwestern Virginia, chain saws were particularly popular with thieves.

As the drug's abuse intensified, so did its casualties. Every week during the spring of 2000, more and more people walked into the Addiction Education Center looking for help in getting off Oxys. Others were being brought into Lee County Hospital on stretchers suffering from overdoses. Most of the hospitalized were teenagers or young adults, some with golf-ball-sized abscesses on their arms, a sign they were shooting up the drug with hypodermic needles.

By early April, Vince Stravino, a younger physician who

worked with Art Van Zee, decided that he had seen enough. He called the headquarters of Purdue, in Stamford, Connecticut, to report the incidents. His call was routed to a physician on the company's staff.

"We are having bad problems," Stravino said. "We are having withdrawals. This is terrible. This is a horrible problem."

The Purdue doctor said she was surprised to hear that people were abusing the drug and assured Stravino she would look into his complaint.

The company filed a required report ten months later notifying the FDA about Stravino's phone call. It read in part:

> Physician reports that unidentified patients (children, teenagers and adults) using OxyContin (controlled-release oxycodone hydrochloride) for unknown reasons "come to the hospital with overdoses and abscesses because of injections." Reportedly, children in the area are "crushing, snorting and injecting OxyContin." Additional information is being requested.

Purdue's report to the FDA also made reference to a follow-up phone call from Stravino that came two months after his first one:

> Additional information received on 05JUN00 from the reporting physician identifies one patient, a 15-year-old Caucasian male who illegally obtained OxyContin 40 mg. tablets. Reportedly, on "07APR00, the patient took an

unknown amount of OxyContin and was found unable to walk, talk coherently at school." Reportedly, the events ended the same date and the patient had a complete recovery. At the time of this report, the patient is undergoing "in-patient treatment." The reporting physician determined that the events were "definitely" related to OxyContin.

For his part, Art Van Zee still was having a hard time coming to grips with the havoc unfolding around him. Through much of that spring he remained focused on the same public health problems in Lee County that had long been his areas of interest, such as teenage pregnancies and infant nutrition. But his concerns about OxyContin were also slowly growing. Van Zee liked research and numbers, so he told a young medical student that he thought it would be a good idea to conduct a survey at Lee High that would ask students about their use of tobacco, alcohol, and both legal and illicit drugs.

One morning, Van Zee's wife, Sue Ella Kobak, was sitting at the family's dining room table when her husband and the medical student who had been staying with the couple walked in. Both men were agitated and talking very fast and Van Zee began to pace in and out of the kitchen.

"Just look at this," he said to Sue Ella, looking shaken. "What do you think this means?"

It was the survey results from Lee High. They showed that 28 percent of all the eleventh graders and 20 percent of twelfth graders said they had tried OxyContin.

It was then that Van Zee understood that something new was happening in his small corner of Appalachia—something beyond the bad things that always seemed to happen there, the problems with joblessness, tough family life, alcohol, and drugs that seemed to flow from one generation to the next. Still, he couldn't understand why.

Then, in May, Vince Stravino, a big soccer fan, flew to Boston to see a game. One day he picked up a copy of the *Boston Globe* and stood transfixed as he read an article in the newspaper about the rampant abuse of a new painkiller in Maine.

The article reported that the drug, OxyContin, was for sale virtually everywhere in rural Washington County, in the state's northern tip. People were traveling hundreds of miles to con prescriptions from doctors by complaining about back pain or migraines. The area had once been a place where people had left their doors unlocked, but now crime was surging and drug treatment centers were being overrun. The situation had reached such a crisis that the local U.S. Attorney had written to doctors throughout the state warning them to be vigilant when prescribing OxyContin.

To Stravino, it all mirrored what was happening in southwestern Virginia. As soon as he got back to Pennington Gap, he showed the article to Van Zee.

"Art, check this out," he said. "This is exactly what is happening here."

Chapter Two

SENIOR NIGHT

AS THE SUMMER OF 2000 drew to a close, Art Van Zee felt as though a lifetime of work was suddenly being swept away. Ever since he had started practicing in Lee County, Van Zee always had a few patients who were abusing one pill or another. But now it was a rare day when he wasn't pulled aside by someone seeking help for a loved one whose desperate addiction to OxyContin was financially or emotionally destroying a family.

In Dryden, the tiny community where Van Zee lived, the son of one of his patients was shot dead, apparently while trying to steal OxyContin from someone else's home. In St. Charles, the town where he worked, escorts accompanied elderly women returning home from church to protect them from walking in on a burglar. Both inside and outside his clinic, Van Zee listened to a parade of horror stories. Families were seeing their life's savings drained by a son's drug habit. Others were scouring pawnshops searching for family heirlooms hocked by an addicted daughter. Meanwhile, Lee County's jail was swelling with young people arrested for drug-related crimes; before long even the nephew of the local sheriff joined their ranks.

These days when Van Zee came home from work, he'd eat a quick dinner and disappear downstairs into the basement. He and his son, Ben, had once played a lot of Ping-Pong down there. But now when his wife, Sue Ella, checked on Art she'd find him sitting in his makeshift home office scanning the Internet for news stories about OxyContin or swapping e-mail messages with other doctors, addiction counselors, and newspaper reporters to try and find out as much as he could about the painkiller.

Sue Ella began to worry about Art. She knew he could withdraw into himself at times, even to the point of depression. Before their marriage in 1986, Van Zee had had a few long-term relationships with women, but none of them stuck. Then Sue Ella, a high-spirited and brassy woman, had decided to make Art her cause.

Sue Ella was a child of Appalachia. She was born in a tiny eastern Kentucky community known as Poor Bottom Hollow. Hers was a breech birth that ripped her hip out of its socket, displacing it. There wasn't a doctor around and her parents didn't expect Sue Ella to make it through the night, so they wrapped her up and placed her behind a warm stove in order to make her as comfortable as possible.

Sue Ella survived the night but her hip wasn't treated; she would grow up walking with a limp. Though her parents had limited educations, both were local activists. Her father, Jake, was a miner and a union official. Her mother, Edith, didn't let a political controversy go by without getting involved. Sue Ella had followed in their footsteps. In the 1960s she worked in the antipoverty program known as Volunteers in Service to America, or VISTA for short, and that was where she met her first husband, John Douglas Kobak. He had dropped out of Harvard University to come to Appalachia as a VISTA volunteer. They fell in love, but John Kobak died suddenly in 1970 at the age of twenty-five while Sue Ella was pregnant with their son, Zeke.

In 1978, while recuperating from an operation to replace her battered hip, she rethought her life. She had long dreamed of becoming a lawyer; not just any lawyer but the kind that would use the law to help make Appalachia a little better. A fear of failing had always stopped her, but not long after her surgery Sue Ella entered law school at the University of Kentucky. When she graduated she quickly went into practice as a community lawyer.

For a time she and Art worked two sides of the same street, their paths frequently crossing. While he attended the sick, she took on coal companies and landfill operators on behalf of local community and environmental groups and worked as well as a public defender, representing criminal defendants who couldn't afford a lawyer. She regularly suggested to Art that he call her. He'd quietly smile and say he might, but never did. A mutual friend suggested to both of them that they go out together. That didn't work either. Two years slipped by. Then one night in 1983, while at a restaurant celebrating a courthouse victory with friends, Sue Ella caught sight of Art as he walked in. She was tipsy from the cheap champagne. "Why haven't you called me yet?" she demanded. Three weeks later he did, and they soon married. Five years after their son Ben was born in 1988, they adopted a daughter, Sophie Mae.

Family life had mellowed Art Van Zee. Though he remained dedicated to the St. Charles clinic, he took days off so he could spend more time with his kids. But now he was spending long hours in his basement office, obsessively trying to put together the pieces of what was happening with OxyContin. The painkiller seemed to be taking a haphazard, irrational journey. Reports about its abuse would suddenly flare up in one area. Then, while that fire was still burning, the spark would jump and land hundreds of miles away, igniting yet another blaze. By the spring of 2000, Van Zee had learned from news reports about the painkiller's abuse not only in Maine and Virginia but also in Florida, Louisiana, Ohio, Pennsylvania, North Carolina, and even Alaska. A law enforcement official in New Orleans told the *Times-Picayune* that OxyContin was being discovered both by people who had abused traditional painkillers such as Vicodin as well as by heroin addicts.

"This probably will be your new Vicodin," that drug agent

was quoted as saying. "Many of our Vicodin abusers are just learning about it. Heroin addicts are starting to use it as a substitute" for heroin.

Locally, a group known as the Lee Coalition for Health turned its attention to figuring out how to deal best with the county's growing OxyContin crisis. Its members included doctors like Van Zee and Vince Stravino, drug abuse counselors like Beth Davies, and law enforcement officials like the sheriff of Lee County, Gary Parsons.

From the start, Stravino was convinced he was witnessing the unfolding of a public health catastrophe. The way Stravino saw it, word about OxyContin's pure and powerful high would just keep spreading along the underground drug grapevine from one satisfied user to another. That's the way it had happened with other prescription drugs that caught on with abusers. But this time, Stravino believed, the dangers were far greater. Because of its supercharged strength, OxyContin could also be less forgiving than those other drugs; as more people experimented with it, a lot of them wouldn't be able to walk away. Instead, Stravino thought, they would get hooked, hurt, or even killed.

Stravino, then thirty-seven years old, was something of an odd man out in Lee County. He'd gone to high school in the industrial city of Bethlehem, Pennsylvania, and had retained both his urban skepticism and his impulsiveness. After graduating from Princeton, Stravino kicked around for a few years, working as a sports reporter on a small-town newspaper, among other jobs. He first encountered Art Van Zee in 1992 when he decided, after entering medical school, that he wanted to get involved in the National Health Service Corps, an arm of the federal Public Health Service that sends doctors to poorer areas throughout the United States. Stravino spent that summer working for Van Zee and became devoted to him, returning periodically to Lee County to work alongside the older doctor as he advanced through his medical training. In 1999, Stravino had come back again, this time as a Public Health Service doctor filling out his remaining obligation to the federal government, which had paid for part of his medical education. Unlike Van Zee, however, Stravino didn't plan to stay for much more than a year. Though he was an outdoor sports enthusiast, he had sophisticated tastes in literature that few people in Lee County shared. Stravino was also single, and he feared that if he remained in Lee County he might stay that way.

As far as he was concerned, there was only one way to solve the OxyContin problem: the Lee Coalition needed to apply pressure on the FDA to take the painkiller off the market. After all, the drug had already created more damage than some medications that the FDA had recalled and there were other painkillers that could be used in its place that posed fewer risks, he told Van Zee.

"This is the way you should do it," he insisted. "There is no other way."

Van Zee thought otherwise. It was clear to him that the drug wasn't some type of pharmaceutical flimflam; it worked, and there were patients with severe, chronic pain whose lives were the better for it. Still, there were things he found troubling. Through his research on the Internet and elsewhere, he'd picked up information about Purdue's efforts to encourage doctors to prescribe OxyContin. Like other drug companies, it had handed out promotional giveaways to doctors, nurses, and others. The small gifts included stuffed animals and beach hats emblazoned with the drug's logo as well as a compact disc entitled *Swing Is Alive*. The cover of the recording, which featured songs like the Andrews Sisters doing "Boogie Woogie Bugle Boy," showed an older couple dancing, free of arthritic pain, apparently after taking OxyContin.

It wasn't the handouts themselves that bothered Van Zee. What disturbed him was that in promoting one of the most powerful narcotics ever sold, Purdue was employing the same marketing strategies used for run-of-the-mill medications. It struck him as particularly ill-advised given the signs of the painkiller's widening abuse.

It wasn't Van Zee's style, however, to point fingers. He believed that the doctors and scientists working at Purdue were decent, well-intentioned professionals who were trying to help people, not hurt them. And if anything, he thought, they probably didn't realize how much chaos OxyContin was causing in a place like Lee County. To him, it seemed that if he could only connect with someone at the company, a fellow doctor perhaps, then they could work together to solve the problem.

Van Zee didn't know anybody at Purdue. But in newspaper articles he had begun to see the name of a company physician,

J. David Haddox, defending OxyContin on the drugmaker's behalf. That August, Van Zee decided to write to Haddox. In that letter he wrote:

> The extent and prevalence of the problem is hard to over-emphasize. . . . These problems are enormous ones for a poor rural area such as ours with minimal resources for dealing with treatment and recovery of hard core narcotic addiction. This also presents an enormous challenge to all in the pain management community, as well as to the Purdue Frederick Company. I would look forward to having a dialogue with you further about this.

At the time Art Van Zee didn't realize it, but his "dialogue" with Purdue had just begun.

By the time Van Zee mailed his letter to Purdue, more than a year had passed since Lindsay Myers had tried her first Oxy. The drug had once gotten her blissfully high, but these days she needed it just to feel normal. Not that she looked that way. Lindsay, who used to love to wear pretty clothes and put on makeup, now arrived bleary-eyed at school dressed in sweatpants and a sweatshirt. Her weight had dropped from 115 pounds to 95, and she looked emaciated. One friend was so upset by Lindsay's appearance that she called her to make sure that everything was okay. When the girl asked Lindsay if the rumor that she was doing drugs was true, Lindsay cut her off.

Other kids at Lee High were less delicate. One day as she walked by, someone shouted out in a singsong voice: "Look at that Lindsay Myers. . . . She is doing drugs. . . . Rich little Lindsay Myers. . . . Boo-hoo." Lindsay walked on. She couldn't care less about what the kids at Lee High thought.

For a time she had continued to meet with Beth Davies, who was also holding separate counseling sessions with Jane Myers. Lindsay thought she had tricked Beth into thinking she was off Oxys. Davies, however, wasn't fooled. Neither was her mother, Jane, though she didn't know what to do. Beth had a lot of sympathy for Jane; she knew that she was struggling to deal with Lindsay without much help from her husband. The nun had worked with lots of parents like her. Naturally, they all wanted to believe that the worst was over and that their child, if just given the right nudge, would soon reappear unchanged and unscathed. But Beth knew that both Jane and Lindsay were in the middle of a situation that, if left unchecked, would get worse.

Beth believed that the only way to rein in Lindsay was to start making her pay for her defiance. She kept telling Jane that the way things stood, Lindsay had nothing to fear. So she kept urging Jane to start drawing lines in the sand: to tell Lindsay that she couldn't stay out late, that she couldn't skip school; the specific issue almost didn't matter. Beth said that the important part was making good on the threat by taking away something that her daughter valued, like her bedroom phone or her Jeep. Otherwise, Lindsay would just continue to run wild. Jane thought Beth was right, but confronting Lindsay wasn't easy;

she had rarely ever said no to her daughter and she felt that doing so now was punishing her for a problem that wasn't her fault.

Eventually, Beth threw up her hands. At one session she told Lindsay that she knew she was lying about not using drugs and that there wasn't any point in meeting again until she decided she wanted help. Lindsay appeared shocked by Beth's directness. Finally, she started talking. The Oxys were robbing all her energy, she said. She also didn't want to be a cheerleader anymore.

"So why are you doing it?" Beth asked.

"Because my mother wants me to," Lindsay said.

"We need to get together," Beth told her. "You need to talk to your mother about this."

But Lindsay decided she didn't want to and soon she stopped seeing Beth. Jane sent her to other addiction counselors. She was just hoping to keep Lindsay's problems quiet and in check so she could get her daughter through her last year of high school. Then, she believed that everything would be okay again; Lindsay could get away from Pennington Gap, go off to college, and start a new life. The drug problem, Jane thought, would sort itself out.

But whether Jane wanted to admit it or not, Lindsay's drug use was already public knowledge. One day in the fall of 2000, a teacher who worked as the coach for Lee High's cheerleading squad called Jane and asked point-blank if it was true that Lindsay was doing drugs. Jane was momentarily shocked into silence. But then she realized that if Lindsay was kicked off the squad, her last link to her old life would be broken.

Jane wasn't about to set her daughter adrift. So she exploded at the woman, accusing her of colluding with the mother of another girl competing with Lindsay to be captain of the squad by spreading lies. Jane said that no one deserved to be captain more than Lindsay; as the only girl on the squad who had been a cheerleader since her freshman year, she had earned it. She also threatened to report the woman's phone call to officials at Lee High. Shortly afterward, the woman quit as the squad's coach and Lindsay was elected captain.

Dealing with Lindsay's new boyfriend proved a lot harder. Lindsay had met Ray, a mechanic who repaired motorcycles and all-terrain vehicles, a year earlier, and before long they were scoring Oxys and driving up Skaggs Hill Road to do them. At the time, Ray was twenty-five, eight years older than Lindsay.

By the time Lindsay and Ray started hanging out together, the teens of Pennington Gap no longer needed to go to Shorty's house to score Oxys. Dealers were now hanging out on just about every street corner on the town's three-block-long downtown strip. If a dealer held up two fingers, that meant that 20-milligram-strength Oxys were for sale; four fingers meant the dealer had the 40-milligram version of the painkiller.

At first, Lindsay didn't say a word to her mother about Ray. But one evening, as Jane was driving past Hardee's, she saw her daughter seated inside her Jeep next to Ray. Jane didn't know Ray well at the time but she was leery of his reputation. She swerved her Mercedes into the Hardee's parking lot and pulled up in front of the Jeep so that it was blocked off. Then she yelled at Lindsay and told her to follow her home.

When they talked, Lindsay insisted that Ray was just a friend. But a few weeks later Lindsay told Jane she was going to a party up on Skaggs Hill Road that some high school friends were giving. That night, the phone rang at the Myerses' house and a caller who wouldn't give her name told Jane that Lindsay was at the party with Ray and that they had been going out with each other. Jane became enraged. She got into her car and started driving as fast as she could, following Skaggs Hill Road until she came to a farmhouse with dozens of cars parked outside its gate. A group of parents was standing guard outside to make sure that kids weren't driving home drunk from the party.

"Is Lindsay Myers here?" Jane asked.

One man said he had seen Lindsay arrive but told Jane that the party was not at the farmhouse, but actually in a field about a half-mile back.

"I'm going to get her," Jane said. "She is with a guy on drugs."

"I'll take you," he told her, opening the door of his pickup.

They bounced along a rutted, dirt road until a bonfire came into view. The bright flames silhouetted dozens of kids dancing to music booming out of a portable CD player. The pickup stopped and Jane jumped out. In the darkness and the fire's glare, Jane could hardly see. She bumped into kids as they danced. "Have you seen Lindsay?" she asked. "Have you seen

Lindsay?" Finally, someone pointed to a girl standing no more than three feet away.

"Mom, what are you doing here?" Lindsay demanded.

Jane grabbed her daughter's arm and started pulling her toward the pickup truck.

"Get in the car and don't make a scene," Jane warned her.

On the way home, the two argued. Jane told Lindsay she didn't want her to see Ray again. Lindsay was defiant.

"I really like him," she told her mother. "I'm going to date him whether you like him or not."

By the start of Lindsay's senior year, she and Ray were together just about all the time. Their Oxy habit was costing about $300 a day. When there was nothing left in Lindsay's bank account, she found another source of cash: the fireproof safe in her parents' bedroom. Lindsay knew where the key was hidden. One day, while she was alone in the house, she took the key and opened the safe. Two cans that looked like shaving cream containers sat on one shelf. She picked up one of the cans and unscrewed the false bottom. Fistfuls of crumpled hundred-dollar bills were stuffed inside. "Oh yeah, thank you, God," she thought, as she began pulling out money. Soon she was stealing money from the safe on a regular basis. Then one day, when she went for the key, she discovered someone had moved it.

The cutoff of Lindsay's cash supply coincided with the Senior Night football game. Senior Night was a long tradition at Lee High, an annual event that took place during the Generals' last home game of the season. At halftime, the name of each player or cheerleader graduating that spring was announced over a loudspeaker. One by one, each senior would then walk, accompanied by his or her proud parents, across the 50-yard line at Five Star Stadium to the applause of two thousand friends and neighbors.

That afternoon, at a pep rally in the school's auditorium, Lindsay and the other cheerleaders stood on stage stomping, twirling, dancing, and screaming at the top of their lungs. This Senior Night was supposed to be Lindsay's night to shine; she was the graduating captain of the cheerleading squad. But as she stood before her classmates, she felt more like a drug-addled rock star performing before an audience of kids straight out of the Brady Bunch. All day she had been running back and forth to the bathroom to throw up or because of diarrhea. Her body throbbed with flulike spasms. She hadn't had an Oxy for twenty-four hours. By now she knew enough about drug withdrawal to realize that she wasn't going to feel right until she got one.

It was right after the pep rally that she met up with Ray. He was out of money but he promised to call his brother in Pennsylvania and beg him to wire $100 right away. As soon as he got the money, he'd buy two Oxy 40s and bring Lindsay one.

A few hours later the game started. The Generals were playing a team from the nearby town of Gate City. Gate City scored first and Lindsay tried to cheer on the Generals while she fought off her growing sickness. She kept scanning the stadium, hoping for a glimpse of Ray. But when the halftime whistle blew, he still hadn't arrived. She saw her parents standing by the sidelines, waiting for the Senior Night ceremony to start. They looked happy and relaxed as they chatted with other parents. It was also a big night for them; pretty soon Lindsay would be moving on.

Not long after the seniors began their procession, Lindsay heard her name boom over the stadium's public address system. "Lindsay Myers is a senior and is the captain of the girls' varsity cheerleading team," the announcer said. "She is the daughter of Jane and Johnny Myers. She is seventeen years old." Jane and Johnny escorted Lindsay across the field. She felt miserable. Once they reached the other sideline, her parents kissed her and told her how proud they were. She waited for them to go and started searching again for Ray.

Finally, she saw him working his way down the stadium steps toward the field. Once he reached it, he walked along the edge of the field near where Lindsay and the other cheerleaders were standing. He didn't make eye contact with her. Instead, Ray kept walking toward a tunnel that ran underneath the stadium. Lindsay waited a few minutes before slipping away from the other cheerleaders to follow him. Ray was waiting in the tunnel; she could see he was already high. He handed her a small cellophane packet with an Oxy 40 inside. She went into a nearby bathroom, where she used a Chapstick to crush it and then snorted the powder. She wiped her nose and ran back out onto the field.

In the late summer of 2000, a few months before the Senior Night game, a letter landed on Art Van Zee's desk. It contained an invitation to a September meeting of a group that called itself the Appalachian Pain Foundation. Van Zee hadn't heard of the organization, but it was clear from the enclosed material that the group's mission was to advocate the aggressive use of strong narcotics to treat patients with significant, recurring pain.

In a cover letter, a physician named Susan Bertrand quoted Thomas Sydenham, a seventeenth-century English apothecary, as having written: "Among the remedies which it has pleased Almighty God to give man to relieve his suffering, none is so universal or efficacious as opium."

The reference was a symbolic one, an emblem of a sea change in medical practice that had led during the 1990s to a sharp rise in the use of powerful, opium-like painkillers. During that decade, proponents of a growing initiative that came to be known as the pain management movement had argued that doctors often withheld such drugs from patients because of misplaced and outdated fears about abuse and addiction. As a result, those experts said, a far greater medical enemy than drug abuse had been created—one they labeled the "undertreatment" of patient pain.

In her letter, Susan Bertrand, who described herself as the founder of the Appalachian Pain Foundation, said the group had recently been formed to help spread this new medical thinking about more aggressively managing pain. It planned a series of meetings to educate doctors about using narcotics frequently in pain treatment as well as to help them discriminate between real patients and drug abusers feigning pain to obtain pills. David Haddox, the Purdue executive, was the principal speaker at those events, and the Connecticut drug company was listed as their sponsor. In the fall of 2000, David Haddox was forty-eight years old and held an impressive array of medical and professional credentials. He was a tall, bearded, fit-looking man with a downturned mouth who had originally gone to dental school. But upon completing his degree he decided instead to become a doctor and eventually received training in pain management, addiction medicine, and psychiatry. During the early 1990s he headed the pain management department at Emory Medical College in Atlanta and also served for a time as the head of the American Academy of Pain Medicine, a small professional group of pain care specialists.

Haddox was also one of the pain management movement's most vocal advocates. While not a researcher, he had helped formulate a concept that had been adopted as one of the movement's catchwords. In a 1989 paper, Haddox and his coauthor had used the term *pseudoaddiction* to describe a condition in which a patient might be mistakenly identified by a doctor as a drug addict because he or she exhibited the common signs of compulsive drug-seeking behavior, like going to multiple doctors to get different prescriptions for narcotics. However, they argued that such actions might actually reflect the desperate plight of a patient who was not being adequately medicated. Such cases of pseudoaddiction would quickly resolve themselves when that patient's pain was treated, Haddox and his coauthor had written.

Haddox's theory was based more on common sense than on statistics; his study was actually just a case report reflecting the behavior of a single patient. Some researchers questioned the extent of pseudoaddictions. But pain care advocates and drug-makers like Purdue championed the concept, elevating it as an equal concern to true addiction because it fit squarely with the view that unwarranted medical fears about narcotics had caused pain patients needless suffering and stigmatization.

During the mid-1990s, Haddox had unsuccessfully sought a job in the pharmaceutical industry. But while giving a talk in 1999 he was approached by a Purdue executive who offered him a position with the drugmaker. He soon became the company's public point man on the issue of OxyContin abuse. The position gave him a high-profile platform to air his strong views about pain care. It also afforded him a channel to exercise his strong and often combative personality.

Haddox had contacted the U.S. Attorney in Maine in March 2000, about a month after newspapers there reported that the prosecutor had alerted state physicians about growing abuse of OxyContin. Three months later, a reporter at a small news-paper in southwestern Virginia received a call from Haddox as well. The paper, the *Richlands News-Press*, had started running articles about an explosion of OxyContin abuse in Tazewell County, Virginia, a county near the West Virginia border about a hundred miles northeast of Pennington Gap. The reporter, Theresa M. Clemons, said that Haddox told her he was calling from Washington, D.C. He had just received a copy of her article by fax, he said, and he wanted to help her put the issues into perspective.

In a subsequent article by Clemons in the Richlands paper,

Haddox was quoted as saying that while misuse or abuse of drugs like OxyContin did occur, such problems were minor compared to the lack of proper pain treatment, and that powerful painkillers like OxyContin posed little addiction threat to patients.

"If you take the medicine like it is prescribed," he said, "the risk of addiction when taking an opioid is one-half of 1 percent."

For Purdue, the newspaper reports in Maine and Virginia had come at an awkward time. By 2000, OxyContin was a blockbuster drug with annual sales of $1 billion, and its future growth appeared limitless. The painkiller had transformed once-sleepy Purdue into an emerging giant, but with about 80 percent of the drugmaker's revenue in 2000 coming from OxyContin's sales, company officials now faced a threat to that success.

The Appalachian Pain Foundation was apparently one of Purdue's first public responses to the abuse of OxyContin. The idea for the group had come from Susan Bertrand, the pain doctor who practiced in the small town of Princeton, West Virginia. But the organization never would have existed without Purdue, which didn't publicize its role in the foundation's birth. As it turned out, Bertrand, who gave paid speeches on Purdue's behalf, had given a talk in early 2000 at a local pharmacy school about pain management. Several Purdue sales reps attended the gathering, and, after her talk, Bertrand went over and sat down with them. She was concerned that the growing abuse of OxyContin in the region might affect the ability of legitimate patients to get the drug. "I was tired of seeing my miners and loggers forced to go from pillar to post," she later said.

She described her idea to the Purdue reps for a group that could act as a vehicle to both advocate the use of strong, long-acting narcotics like OxyContin in pain treatment and help doctors understand how better to use them. The reps welcomed the plan and told her that Purdue would pay for the foundation's costs, such as meeting hall rentals, and that they would take care of the administrative chores like inviting doctors to the group's meetings.

By this time Purdue needed a voice outside itself in Appalachia. The company was aware that several doctors in the region were already under scrutiny or criminal investigation for illegally prescribing OxyContin and other powerful narcotics, while other physicians, uncomfortable with the growing publicity about the painkiller, were pulling back from prescribing it. Oxy-Contin had even gotten a nickname. Some newspaper writers had started calling it "hillbilly heroin."

In August 2000 a contingent of Purdue executives including David Haddox arrived in Charleston, West Virginia, for the kickoff meeting of the Appalachian Pain Foundation. Haddox was the main speaker at the gathering, which was billed as a pain treatment seminar for local doctors. But before the event started, the Purdue team met briefly with a contingent of officials from Tazewell County, the area featured in the *Richlands News-Press* articles, who had driven up to Charleston that day to tell the company executives about the problems that Oxy-Contin was causing.

Years later, Dennis Lee, the prosecutor for Tazewell County, would recall painting a vivid picture for David Haddox and the others of the devastating toll that OxyContin misuse was taking in terms of addiction and crime. However, Lee later said he walked away from that discussion feeling that neither Haddox nor his colleagues had fully grasped the severity of the crisis. They had been extremely sympathetic, but they had also said they believed that cases like the ones in Tazewell County were isolated. Haddox and the others also suggested that the problems being seen with OxyContin in Appalachia and northern Maine were possibly linked by socioeconomic factors. Both areas, the Purdue executives noted, had high unemployment rates and a long history of using narcotic painkillers to treat injuries caused by regional occupations like farming, mining, and logging.

One month later, in September, Art Van Zee, Beth Davies, and Elizabeth Vines piled into Van Zee's car and drove to Southwest Virginia Community College, located near the town of Richlands, where the Appalachian Pain Foundation was holding its next meeting. Again, David Haddox was the event's main speaker, and Van Zee, having already written to the Purdue executive, figured that he couldn't pass up a chance to meet him.

During his talk Haddox emphasized, as he always did, that doctors had to take precautions when prescribing drugs like OxyContin, precautions such as monitoring a patient's use of such pills and keeping accurate records. But as Van Zee sat listening to Haddox and Susan Bertrand talk, he worried that

Purdue was promoting greater use of powerful narcotics at a time when OxyContin's abuse in southwestern Virginia was out of control.

Tazewell County prosecutor Dennis Lee was also at the Richlands meeting, and both he and Van Zee spoke during a panel discussion about the catastrophes affecting their communities.

"We have never seen anything like this before," Lee was quoted by the *Roanoke Times* as saying. "There is just no comparison."

When the Richlands meeting ended, Van Zee approached Haddox and introduced himself as the doctor who had recently written to him. He first commended Purdue for its interest in seeing the misuse of its drug reduced, but then he told Haddox that he was concerned that the company was still sending out promotional gimmicks like the Swing Era music CD.

"How is that any different from what every other drug company does?" Haddox responded.

"People aren't stealing from their families or breaking into their neighbors' homes over blood pressure pills," Van Zee said.

Haddox got ready to leave; he had a drive ahead. The following morning he was scheduled to give a talk under the Appalachian Pain Foundation's banner to doctors in eastern Kentucky, another area rife with OxyContin abuse. He suggested that Van Zee direct his complaints elsewhere.

"I don't have anything to do with that," Van Zee would later recall Haddox saying. "That is a marketing department issue."

A WAR AGAINST PAIN

THE MOVEMENT TO treat pain more aggressively with powerful narcotics like OxyContin had only just begun in 1981 when a physician who'd emerge as its scientific superstar walked into the Albert Einstein College of Medicine to begin his medical residency. That doctor, whose name is Russell K. Portenoy, had originally been interested in behavioral neurology, the treatment of illnesses and injuries affecting the brain. But Portenoy, who was then twenty-six, didn't realize that day that his medical career was about to head in a new direction.

As he was introduced to the Bronx Hospital's teaching staff, Portenoy asked about their medical specialties. One of them,

Dr. Ronald Kanner, said his focus was pain treatment. Portenoy smiled at Kanner, thinking he was joking.

"You can't do pain," he said. "Pain isn't a disease. It's a symptom."

Two decades later, Russell Portenoy would rank among this country's most respected specialists in the treatment of severe chronic pain and be the leading advocate for the use of strong, long-lasting narcotics in its treatment. His reputation as an innovative researcher and thinker would grow so quickly that a major New York City hospital, the Beth Israel Medical Center, would create a pain department in order to lure him there. Between 1981 and 2001, Portenoy wrote or coauthored more than 145 scientific articles about pain treatment and contributed to fifteen books. His confidence and quick, easy wit made him a popular speaker at scientific conferences and medical conventions and a sought-after consultant with pharmaceutical companies that were producing and marketing pain medications. He was frequently quoted in newspaper and magazine articles about pain and appeared on television programs on the subject. Twenty years after his career began, the demands on Portenoy's time were so great that new pain patients often waited four months for an appointment.

Those who made it through Portenoy's doors typically inhabited a particular circle of hell known as chronic, nonmalignant pain, or intense pain from causes other than cancer. Severe, ongoing pain often accompanies cancer, as growing malignant tumors press against sensitive nerves or destroy bone. Recurring episodes of serious pain can also be hallmarks of diseases such as sickle-cell anemia, diabetes, rheumatoid arthritis, and shingles. But for many of Portenoy's patients, pain thrived as though it had a life of its own, outlasting the injury or illness that had first caused it. In the face of treatment, it often proved resistant, or *intractable*. It was as if the nervous systems of Portenoy's patients had gone haywire and had begun spewing out a constant stream of pain messages.

In some patients, a minor injury like a twisted ankle or the breaking of a tiny wrist bone might cause a leg or an arm to swell, sweat, discolor, and even become palsied. In other patients, severe pain might leap from limb to limb without apparent reason, as though playing a game of hide-and-seek. Some patients experience bolts of "phantom pain" seemingly emanating from a limb long severed from their body. Others are rendered nauseous, speechless, or prostrate by migraine headaches, cluster headaches, or trigeminal neuralgia, a condition in which intense, ripping pain sporadically explodes along major facial nerves. Still other patients awake from surgery or even a minor procedure like a cosmetic facelift to find themselves accompanied from that day forward by intense burning pain, apparently because a doctor's scalpel had nicked a nerve.

The lives of many sufferers become consumed by a single idea: finding relief. In 1989, Anthony Guaimano suddenly started to experience facial pains while working as a school custodian in Jersey City, New Jersey. Guaimano, thinking that the problem was temporary, would take aspirin at first or retreat to the school's bathroom where he massaged his face or applied hot and cold compresses. But the episodes continued, and the pain, which started on the right side of his face and traveled across it, intensified to the point of being unbearable.

Soon, a decade-long medical odyssey began. One doctor gave Guaimano blood pressure medication; another doctor gave him lithium, a drug prescribed for manic-depression. He received migraine treatments. He also began taking fistfuls of narcotic painkillers like Percocet. His condition worsened to the point that he was forced to stop working. Eventually, one doctor suggested that Guaimano might be able to abort the attacks by breathing in oxygen, so he began to travel everywhere with the type of small, portable oxygen tank that emphysema sufferers use. When he felt an attack coming on, Guaimano would press a thumb against the right side of his face and close one nostril with a finger while breathing in oxygen. It helped, but his misery was still such that he considered a dentist's recommendation to have some of his teeth removed.

Guaimano's son thought his father might be suffering from trigeminal neuralgia, the sporadic and excruciating facial pain condition, and even flew from his home in California to attend a conference in Philadelphia about the problem. There he heard about a Pittsburgh physician who was claiming success with a surgical approach to the condition. Not long afterward, Guaimano and his wife loaded his oxygen tanks into a car and drove out to Pittsburgh from their New Jersey home. After examining Guaimano, however, that doctor told him that he couldn't help him; he was suffering not from trigeminal neuralgia but rather from cluster headaches, a syndrome of unknown cause that often affects middle-aged men and produces intense pain episodes.

Frustrated again, Guaimano and his wife returned home. One day she saw a television documentary about pain that featured Russell Portenoy. They managed to get an appointment with Portenoy, who put Guaimano on a strong dose of OxyContin. The painkiller seemed to work like a charm for Guaimano, and during one visit he sang its praises to the pain specialist; he seemed overjoyed by the prospect of getting his life back.

OxyContin didn't work as well for all of Portenoy's patients. But Portenoy was a strong believer in the value of long-acting narcotics to treat chronic pain, and there were similar drugs in his armamentarium. One was fentanyl, a powerful synthetic opioid that was marketed by a unit of Johnson & Johnson in the form of a skin patch under the brand name Duragesic. Another long-acting painkiller was methadone, a substance best known as a maintenance narcotic for heroin addicts that had started its medical life as a pain treatment.

Portenoy, like many pain specialists, also used other pharmaceuticals to supplement or amplify the effects of narcotics; among them, several drugs used to control epilepsy, for instance, effectively helped dampen pain.

For pain patients, an expert of Portenoy's stature was rarely the first stop. By the time he saw a patient they were usually loaded down with years of medical records, stacks of X rays, and reams of diagnostic test results. Sometimes the data provided clues to a patient's condition. But for Portenoy and specialists like him, deciphering pain was like trying to solve a puzzle. The answer was unique to each patient, embedded somewhere within each personal jumble of physical and psychological conditions and social and emotional lives.

"Pain is a little science, a lot of intuition, and a lot of art," Russell Portenoy liked to say.

Pain is frequently described as the most commonplace of medical complaints. It is also the most subjective; ultimately, doctors must rely on patients to describe their pain. Pain can be sharp or dull. It can ache or shoot. It can burn or chill. Some patients describe their pain as mimicking the pounding of a hammer; others as the beating of a drum; still others as the stabbing of a knife. Each person also has his or her own pain threshold, or the point at which he or she experiences pain. There are also cultural aspects to pain's perception. David B. Morris, in his book *The Culture of Pain*, noted that a study performed in the 1950s at a veterans' hospital in San Francisco found that while Jewish and Italian-American patients tended to be uninhibited about expressing pain, patients of Irish or Protestant Anglo-Saxon origin were more tight-lipped.

There is even a small percentage of people who are born insensitive to pain. What may seem like an enviable asset is, in fact, a disastrous condition that can cause one to sit calmly on a scalding radiator oblivious to the fact that he or she is being severely burned. The most widely cited case involved a Canadian girl referred to in reports as Miss C. In their book *The Challenge of Pain*, Dr. Ronald Melzack and Dr. Patrick D. Wall wrote that Miss C's congenital insensitivity to pain caused her as a girl to bite off the tip of her tongue, and that as a young woman she developed severely infected joints because she was able to stand in ways that others would find excruciating. Those afflicted with the condition typically die at a young age; Miss C succumbed to massive infections at twenty-nine.

In many ways it is pain's subjective nature that for so long made it an also-ran in the hierarchy of medical specialties. Physicians like problems that they can diagnose and solve, and pain often doesn't lend itself to that. There is no pain thermometer, no pain gauge, no pain meter. A doctor can't send a patient's blood out hoping to find clues about his or her pain and its intensity. Technology, be it in the form of X ray machines or more advanced devices like MRIs, is sometimes helpful but notoriously unreliable. For instance, while 80 percent of those people who complain of back pain have X rays that show evidence of spinal disc degeneration, about 70 percent of all adults who exhibit similar problems on X rays have no pain. The science of measuring pain had made such little progress by the end of the twentieth century that one of its key tools was a scale of crude cartoonlike faces that ranged from smiling to grimacing, to which patients pointed to indicate their pain's intensity.

The history of pain management as a modern medical specialty reaches back only to 1973, when 350 researchers from around the world gathered near Seattle, Washington, for a meeting that led to the creation of the International Association for the Study of Pain. But for millennia prior to that get-together, physicians, philosophers, priests, and shamans had sought to understand pain and its causes. In its simplest terms, that search has been an effort to understand the roles that the body, the mind, and the emotions play in the cause of pain and its sensation. Many ancient civilizations such as those in Babylonia, Egypt, and India all believed that pain was experienced in the heart and signaled an emotional unbalance or an invasion of the body by evil or mischievous spirits. Later, a Greek scientist named Galen began the first systematic examination of the nervous system. His work, however, was largely forgotten until the Renaissance led to a realization that the brain constantly received pain signals, ignoring some and amplifying others. By the late twentieth century, scientists had unraveled the secrets of the nervous system even further, discovering specific chemicals that transmitted pain as well as others that blocked the sensation of it.

There also have been relatively few advances in pain treatment. Opium, which comes from the opium poppy, was used for thousands of years to both treat pain and produce pleasure. Through much of history, doctors believed that opium was benign, in part because it was the only medicine available to combat life-threatening conditions like uncontrolled diarrhea. In his comprehensive look at the drug's uses and history, Martin Booth wrote in the book *Opium: A History* that during the nineteenth century it was found in a host of preparations like paregoric and laudanum sold to combat a host of medical ills as well as malaise. For example, opium was the basis of so-called soothing solutions, potions given by destitute and over-worked Victorian-era women to quiet their babies so they could get some sleep. The potion was also used on "baby farms," the notorious orphanages of the same period. The opium drinks rendered infants virtually comatose, damaging some for life, Booth wrote.

It was in the early 1800s that chemists discovered that much of opium's painkilling power came from a constituent within it, a substance that they named morphine after Morpheus, the Greek god of sleep. Morphine's use became widespread, eclipsing that of opium in many medical applications. Soon researchers isolated other chemicals from opium, including one called thebaine, the substance that is used as the starting material in the production of oxycodone.

By the mid-nineteenth century, however, it had started to become apparent that the broad use of opiates carried a price. Around 1900 there were an estimated three hundred thousand morphine addicts in the United States alone, including many Civil War veterans who had gotten addicted to the painkiller while being treated for war-related injuries or illnesses. The condition was so commonplace it was called "soldier's disease." Finally, around World War I, the medical profession recognized morphine's intense, habit-forming potential and the term *addiction* was first widely used.

As a result, physicians no longer viewed opiates as benign but rather as substances that carried a high risk of so-called iatrogenic addiction, or addiction induced by a doctor in the course of treating a patient. For example, surveys performed in the 1920s of patients in drug addiction treatment programs estimated that from 9 percent to 24 percent of them had first been exposed to such medications while being treated by a physician for pain.

Doctors had something else to worry about. In 1914, the federal government passed the Harrison Act, the nation's first drug law. It was essentially a taxing and record-keeping statute rather than a law enforcement one. But the U.S. Supreme Court issued an opinion in 1919 that interpreted the Harrison Act as also banning the prescribing of narcotics to those addicted to them. By the late 1930s more than twenty-five thousand doctors had been charged with offenses related to the law.

Physicians still employed morphine to treat severe pain, particularly the intense suffering experienced by cancer patients. But even here, medical views about morphine's addictive potential affected how it was used, resulting for decades in needless agony for thousands of cancer victims.

Until the early 1990s many doctors prescribed morphine to cancer patients on a so-called PRN basis—medical shorthand for *pro re nata*, or "as needed." Morphine's painkilling effect typically lasted for about four hours, so under the PRN approach cancer sufferers were supposed to ask for and receive their next dose of morphine once they felt pain returning. But cancer patients often didn't immediately get another dose of the drug, even when they begged for it or screamed out in agony. Some doctors and nurses faced with a patient's desperate demands didn't hear a cry for help but rather the prevarications of a suspected drug abuser. And because of prevailing medical and social stigmas about narcotics use, some medical professionals, as well as some patients, believed that a stiff upper lip was the right approach to pain. Whatever the reason, cancer pain often escalated to such a severe state that the amount of morphine finally needed to subdue it sucked the patient down into a mental stupor.

It was this horrific situation that provided the genesis for the pain management movement. Dr. Cicely M. Saunders, an English physician, was one of its pioneers. In 1967, Dr. Saunders opened the first facility devoted to the care of those in the final months of life, St. Christopher's in London. Saunders' philosophy was that the terminally ill should die a dignified death, not in a sterile hospital, but rather in comfortable surroundings, even one's home. She also believed that life's end should be as pain-free as possible.

By the early 1980s, the hospice movement that Saunders had started arrived in this country. However, a few American hospitals—most notably Memorial Sloan-Kettering Cancer Center in New York City—had already begun to use morphine more aggressively in cancer care. Experts there believed that a cancer patient should be given morphine routinely, not just when it was asked for, in order to keep the drug's analgesic level constant in the bloodstream and to avoid the roller-coaster effect of the PRN approach. The facility's extensive work with morphine also produced findings of potentially wider significance: contrary to accepted medical expectations, cancer patients who received large morphine doses weren't becoming addicted to the drug or even experiencing the type of euphoric high associated with its abuse.

Over time, the work at Memorial Sloan-Kettering changed the way cancer pain was treated throughout the United States. But it would also highlight what pain experts believed was another pervasive problem in this country—the inadequate treatment of serious pain unrelated to cancer, so-called chronic nonmalignant pain. This diverse group of pain sufferers—those with back pain, arthritis, sickle-cell anemia, and a host of other conditions—made up the vast majority—as many as 80 percent, according to some estimates—of those in constant pain.

In the mid-1980s a variety of methods to treat noncancer pain existed, including surgical procedures, cortisone shots, and alternative approaches such as biofeedback and exercise. But at that time there was also a furious debate raging within the cloistered world of pain treatment about how or even whether narcotics should be used to treat constant pain. In fact, just as Russell Portenoy was starting his career, many leading pain specialists were arguing against it.

Those experts believed that patients with chronic bouts of pain that had no clear origin often suffered from a complex mix of physical, psychological, and emotional problems. And those physicians felt that a steady regimen of painkillers caused some pain patients to become drugged-out zombies, turned others into drug abusers, and often intensified pain rather than relieved it. Several studies of chronic headache patients indicated that those who habitually used narcotics or over-the-counter painkillers, for instance, suffered frequent "rebound" attacks induced by the drugs' apparent suppression of the body's own pain-fighting system.

Those favoring a nonpharmaceutical approach also tended to see some chronic pain patients as head cases; that is, people who used pain complaints as a way to either get out of work, emotionally manipulate others, or obtain drugs. While lower back pain was rarely diagnosed, for example, by doctors prior to World War II, such complaints by the 1980s were the leading cause of chronic pain and accounted, by one estimate, for an astonishing 5 percent of all doctors' visits. This apparent epidemic of lower back pain, some specialists believed, had less to do with nerve problems or physical injuries than with work-related stress and job dissatisfaction. Researchers theorized that unhappy employees, after sustaining a relatively minor injury, preferred to drag out their sick leave rather than return to work, and that their depression and susceptibility to pain deepened the longer they remained home. Large financial awards from juries or compensation boards were seen as added lures. After determining that more than half of a group of pain patients involved in lawsuits had pain rooted in emotional causes rather than physical ones, one researcher dubbed the phenomenon "chronic pain in litigation."

Throughout the 1970s and into the 1980s there had been an emphasis on a so-called multidisciplinary approach to severe pain. Large centers based on this method operated at the University of Washington and the University of Miami. Patients entering such programs dropped their painkillers at the door, sometimes by the shopping bagful. Then they were slowly weaned off narcotics to prevent withdrawal and put through a regimen of programs that emphasized physical therapy, psychotherapy, and other techniques including behavior modification. Many found themselves spending several hours a day doing stretching and strengthening exercises like aerobics and swimming. Since many pain patients suffered from anxiety because they anticipated future attacks, they were also taught relaxation and stress management techniques as substitutes for the addicting tranquilizers they had been taking.

It was into this muddled landscape of views about pain and its treatment that Russell Portenoy stepped at the start of his residency at the Albert Einstein College of Medicine in 1981. He was soon spending his days in the basement office of his newfound mentor, Ronald Kanner. For his part, Kanner was a pain care activist. He had worked at Memorial Sloan-Kettering and believed that many doctors in this country were underutilizing opiate-like drugs because of overwrought fears. One researcher called the attitude American "opiophobia," a term that soon became a rallying cry for the pain management movement.

In Russell Portenoy, Dr. Kanner saw not only an eager acolyte but also the makings of a world-class researcher. So he quickly threw him into the fray, handing him a Bronx telephone book and his first assignment: to start calling area druggists to ask about the different kinds of Schedule II narcotics like morphine, Dilaudid, and Percocet they kept in stock, and the amounts of each. What Portenoy learned was that the druggists had very few narcotic painkillers available because they were rarely prescribed, and small quantities because of robbery fears.

At the same time, doctors at Albert Einstein College started referring their pain patients to Portenoy. In treating them, the young physician got to see pain in its many forms—and the hard time patients often had getting help. One of his patients, a thirty-five-year-old black man, had sickle-cell anemia. He told Portenoy that each time he suffered an attack he was forced to go to a hospital and endure hours of painful waiting before a hospital emergency room doctor gave him a few painkillers. Portenoy wrote him a prescription for Percocet so that the man would have a ready supply at home. When he handed him the prescription, the man broke down and cried; no doctor had ever trusted him before, he said.

In 1984, Portenoy began a research fellowship at Memorial Sloan-Kettering, on Manhattan's Upper East Side. The facility in 1981 had become the nation's first hospital to open a unit specifically devoted to the treatment of patient pain, appointing as its head Dr. Kathleen M. Foley, a seminal figure in the pain field.

Some physicians might have found Memorial Sloan-Kettering a difficult place to work; it was a hospital where many patients made their last, losing stand against cancer. However, Portenoy, who worked as a researcher on Foley's small team, saw his job as one of giving comfort. His role, unlike that of an oncologist, wasn't to fight cancer's progress but to make the lives of its sufferers more bearable.

"We were the white hats," he would say later. "We didn't feel we had to battle the disease. We didn't feel we would have to be defeated. You'd walk into a room with a person with cancer that has metastasized and the family is there in despair. But you'd walk out of the room having done something to help."

Soon, developments took place that changed the field of pain care. In 1984, Purdue Frederick, then a small drug company, began selling a long-acting version of morphine in a timed-release tablet under the brand name MS Contin. Leading cancer pain researchers considered the formulation a breakthrough because a tablet's painkilling effect lasted up to twelve hours, allowing patients to sleep through the night. Because it didn't contain over-the-counter additives like aspirin, doctors could also increase the drug's use as patient pain increased without worrying about side effects like liver damage.

The next big development came from Portenoy. He had already begun to turn his attention beyond cancer patients toward the large sea of patients with all kinds of severe, chronic pain. A report he published in 1986 would serve as the scientific launching pad for the pain management movement to broaden its reach and embrace this larger group. The 1986 report, coauthored by Kathleen Foley, was entitled "Chronic Use of Opioid Analgesics in Non-Malignant Pain." The study was an extremely small one by research standards, involving just thirty-eight Memorial Sloan-Kettering patients with a mix of conditions like chronic back and facial pain. But bearing the imprimatur of Foley and Memorial Sloan-Kettering, its impact was enormous. It also quickly catapulted Portenoy, then only thirty-one, into the role of a scientific luminary within the small sphere of pain care.

At its core, Portenoy's idea was simple and compassionate: he argued that there was a "subpopulation" of chronic pain patients who, having failed to get relief otherwise, might benefit greatly from the long-term use of powerful narcotics, drugs already shown to be safe when used in cancer patients. "We conclude that opioid maintenance therapy can be a safe, salutary and more humane alternative to the options of surgery or no treatment in those patients with intractable non-malignant pain and no history of drug abuse," Portenoy and Foley wrote.

Portenoy soon began to lecture around the country, his talks typically sponsored by drug companies or by the Dannemiller Foundation, an organization supported by the pharmaceutical industry that puts on continuing education programs for physicians. The message he brought was not always a welcome one. Some experts favoring a multidisciplinary strategy to combat pain considered Portenoy an "evangelist" for a drug-based approach. Also, they argued that while Portenoy's use of powerful narcotics had subdued his patients' pain, few of those patients had shown functional improvements.

However, a new generation of pain specialists entering the profession saw it differently. They believed that reducing severe and incessant pain was a laudable goal in itself. As Portenoy's reputation spread, his talks drew ever larger crowds.

"When you are the first person bringing a radical approach,

a lot of people want to hear what you have to say," recalled one pain specialist who attended a Portenoy lecture.

Russell Portenoy's work led to far more than a shift in medical views about the value of strong narcotics in the treatment of pain. It also provided pain management activists with the data and statistics they needed to push their offense ahead on both the political and social fronts.

In a string of scientific papers published beginning in the mid-1980s, Portenoy argued that the high addiction rates noted by researchers in the 1920s were misleading because they reflected a biased population—participants in drug treatment programs. Instead he maintained that when one looked at the experience of pain patients who had received narcotics in medical settings, the addictive risk of such drugs all but disappeared. There was scant data on that subject, but Portenoy pointed to three reports that were quickly adopted by the pain management movement as a kind of holy scientific trinity. In 1980, the *New England Journal of Medicine* published data about narcotics use and addiction in hospital patients. The second study, which appeared in a 1977 issue of the journal, *Headache*, looked at the problem use of narcotic painkillers by chronic sufferers. And the third study, published in *Pain* magazine in 1982, reviewed the experience of burn patients given narcotics while undergoing debridement, an extremely painful procedure in which dead skin is removed.

As characterized by Portenoy and other narcotics advocates,

these three reports suggested that there was minimal, if any, risk of addiction among pain patients who previously hadn't abused drugs. As they saw it, the hospital study found "only four cases of addiction among 11,882 hospitalized patients," while the study of chronic headache sufferers identified only "three problem cases among 2,369 patients." These were the studies behind the claim that narcotics posed an addiction risk of "less than one percent," a figure that Purdue executives such as David Haddox would continue to cite years later even as Oxy-Contin cut its swath of addiction and abuse across places like Lee County.

For his part, Portenoy was careful to note in professional publications that the evidence about the value of long-acting opioids in chronic pain treatment was scanty and did not lend itself to "doctrinaire pronouncements." He also emphasized that doctors had to rigorously examine patients for the potential to abuse, including taking detailed family histories.

"The limited number of controlled trials, combined with disparities and inherent biases of the survey literature, preclude definitive conclusions about the risks and benefits of long-term opioid therapy," he wrote in a paper that appeared in the *Journal of Pain and Symptom Management.*

But most doctors didn't read about Portenoy's work in such highly specialized publications. Instead they learned about it from newspapers, magazines, and television, forums in which Portenoy expressed far less equivocal views.

"There is a growing literature showing that these drugs can be used for a long time, with few side effects, and that addiction and abuse are not a problem," he told the *New York Times* at around the same time that his report in the *Journal of Pain and Symptom Management* appeared.

There was little question in the early 1990s that changes were needed in how pain was treated. According to one estimate, many physicians received only an hour of training in medical school about pain and its management. Also, while the use of strong narcotics for cancer pain was gaining favor, resistance to the drugs' use in other situations continued to run deep. A 1991 University of Wisconsin survey reported, for example, that only 12 percent of state medical board members said they viewed such treatment as acceptable medical practice. The pain treatment of certain groups of patients—in particular the elderly and newborns—continued to border on the barbaric. Up until the mid-1980s, surgeons often operated on desperately ill newborns without using painkillers because they were considered too risky for infants to tolerate. Even after that date children in pain often were inadequately medicated.

"Most adults would be shocked if they saw what was done to children in hospitals without anesthetics," one pediatric pain expert told the *Los Angeles Times* in 1991. "It's like roping and holding down a steer to brand it."

Spurred by the pain management movement, government authorities soon began promoting better pain care. In 1992, for example, a unit of the Public Health Service called the Agency for Health Care Policy issued new guidelines that urged hospitals to use powerful narcotics more aggressively to treat the type of acute pain experienced as the result of surgery. Dr. James O. Mason, the Public Health Service's top official, told the *New York Times* that the new recommendations were needed to dispel "cultural" myths that pain "is necessary to build character, that infants do not feel pain, that elderly patients have a higher pain tolerance, and that narcotics used for postoperative pain are often addictive."

Meanwhile, narcotics advocates also had begun to make slow but steady progress on the state level to encourage a more liberal use of strong painkillers. Beginning in 1989 with Texas, a growing number of states began passing laws or adopting medical board guidelines that specifically recognized the value of powerful narcotics in treating severe intractable pain. Pain care experts had long argued that such new rules were necessary because narcotics agents and medical boards had unfairly targeted doctors who used large amounts of painkillers.

Most advocacy movements need good bogeymen, and pain management activists had long identified their enemy as any law, institution, or regulatory mechanism that they viewed as unduly deterring doctors from prescribing strong narcotics. Along with narcotics agents and medical board members with outdated views, another prominent enemy on their list were the so-called prescription monitoring systems used by some states to track physicians' use of controlled substances.

The purpose of such systems, which existed in the mid-1990s in fourteen states, was to identify doctors whose high prescribing volumes suggested that they might be running illicit medical operations known as "pill mills" or "script mills", where prescriptions were written in exchange for the price of an office visit. States like New York, which in 1977 had started monitoring Schedule II narcotics like morphine and oxycodone, typically adopted the systems in response to outbreaks of prescription drug abuse.

For years, both drug companies and the American Medical Association had fiercely opposed prescription monitoring. But as the pain management movement began to gather force in the early 1990s, it took over a leading role in the fight, arguing that monitoring was having a "chilling effect" on legitimate narcotics prescribing because doctors didn't want to land on the regulatory radar of a state drug enforcement agency.

One leading voice questioning monitoring was David E. Joranson, who headed a think tank at the University of Wisconsin that was initially known as the Pain Treatment Group and was later renamed the Pain and Policies Studies Group. Joranson had been the administrator of Wisconsin's Controlled Substances Board when he became involved in the late 1980s in an initiative to improve cancer pain care in the state. He soon left government and devoted himself to pain care advocacy.

In a series of influential papers that began appearing in the early 1990s, Joranson argued that monitoring was of little proven law enforcement value, and that the hesitancy of doctors in states with monitoring to write narcotics prescriptions was unfairly affecting many innocent patients.

While Joranson publicly stated he favored an approach to monitoring that "balanced" the needs of law enforcement and

pain patients, he and other narcotics activists were often un-
bending. For example, when several states with paper-based
monitoring systems that physicians complained about as bur-
densome advocated moving to simplified, electronic prescribing
systems, Joranson opposed that too. "Requiring the use of these
prescription forms would send an unmistakable message to
physicians that prescribing controlled substances could give
them an unwanted high profile with the police or licensing authorities if they order more than a minimal amount for patients
in pain or suffering from other disorders," Joranson and a coauthor wrote in a 1993 issue of the *American Pain Society Bulletin*.

At the time, some medical experts such as Dr. Sidney Wolfe
of the Health Research Group, an advocacy group often critical
of the pharmaceutical industry, argued that there was little evidence to support the "chilling effect" of prescription monitoring cited by Joranson and others. And they added that
monitoring helped deter inappropriate and illegal prescribing.
Still, the pain management movement had grown strong
enough by the mid-1990s to help defeat a congressional initiative to create a national prescription monitoring system as well
as efforts to create or broaden such programs in some states.

Ultimately, it was the news media that carried the pain management movement's message into the public's consciousness
and the social mainstream. By the mid-1990s, major newspapers
and magazines had begun to routinely publish articles about
pain and its inadequate treatment. For example, within the
space of two months during the spring of 1997, *U.S. News &
World Report* published an article entitled "The Quality of

Mercy," while *Forbes* magazine carried a piece entitled "The Morphine Myth." Leading pain experts such as Russell Portenoy were frequently quoted in such articles, which also trumpeted the data from the three addiction studies cited by Portenoy as showing that narcotics held little if any addiction risk for patients.

Other writers chose to dramatize the battle against pain, drawing sympathetic portraits of pain patients deprived of medications they needed because of medical "myths" about narcotics, intrusive regulations, and meddling government drug agents. One lengthy article in a 1997 issue of *Playboy* magazine suggested that a government frustrated by its losing war against illicit drugs had turned to easier pickings—pain patients and the doctors who cared for them:

> Needing a winnable war, the government had cracked
> down in doctors' offices. Across the country, state agents,
> allied with the DEA, have staked out pain clinics under
> the assumption that wherever narcotics are prescribed,
> diversion of the drugs will soon follow. In pursuing this
> theory, the government has criminalized an entire class of
> patients and scared doctors into abandoning them.

But journalists often missed another part of the story: the drug industry's role in the pain management movement. Industry money supported research by investigators like Kathleen Foley and Russell Portenoy, and virtually every pain management specialist was a consultant or paid speaker for a narcotics producer.

Drug companies subsidized patient advocacy organizations like the American Pain Foundation. Funds from narcotics makers also increasingly poured throughout the 1990s into the American Pain Society and the American Academy of Pain Medicine, the two principal groups representing those doctors specializing in pain treatment. In 1997, for instance, Purdue contributed half a million dollars to underwrite the work of a joint committee formed by the two groups that issued a report that year urging the broader medical use of powerful narcotics. It was headed by David Haddox, who was then in private practice.

Another recipient of industry funds was David Joranson's group at the University of Wisconsin. Some nonprofit organizations like the Robert Wood Johnson Foundation made sizable contributions to the Pain and Policies Study Group. But drugmakers like Janssen Pharmaceuticals, Knoll Pharmaceuticals, and Ortho-McNeil were also among its backers. The biggest industry donor was Purdue Frederick, the maker of MS Contin and, later, OxyContin. Over time, Purdue gave hundreds of thousands of dollars to Joranson's group.

There were also strong ideological ties—ties between narcotics advocates and the pharmaceutical industry that some pain experts would find hard to shake when the public health crisis involving OxyContin exploded in places like southwestern Virginia. Throughout the 1990s, many leading proponents of a more aggressive use of narcotics viewed Purdue not as a profit-seeking enterprise but as an ally in a noble social cause: the betterment of pain treatment through physician and public education.

"I view them as our colleagues in education," Kathleen Foley told one interviewer in 1996. "It was not the government that wanted to educate; it was not the National Cancer Institute that wanted to educate. It was the drug company that wanted to improve pain management."

Still, some experts watched with dismay as the agendas of professional groups like the American Pain Society shifted to reflect a pharmacological approach to treatment. "The A.P.S. should really stand for the American Pharmaceutical Society," said Dennis Turk, a clinical psychologist who specializes in pain treatment.

But the influence of those championing nondrug approaches to chronic pain was fading for other reasons as well. Studies indicated that chronic pain patients who entered multidisciplinary programs at places like the University of Miami emerged improved over time but had high relapse rates. The era of managed care was also in full throttle, and those who treated pain faced the same economic pressures as psychotherapists. Insurers were willing to pay for pills but not for the therapy and rehab regimes offered by multidisciplinary centers that could cost up to $20,000.

As the narcotics bandwagon gathered steam, a few voices of dissent were raised. In a 1996 paper published in the *Journal of Pain and Symptom Management*, Dennis Turk argued that the views of the opposing experts—the multidisciplinary advocates and those favoring opioids—were both mistaken because their perspectives had been molded by small and unique groups of patients. Turk maintained that multidisciplinary disciples unfairly dismissed narcotics because drugs hadn't worked for their patients who presented extremely difficult cases. However, he also cautioned that narcotics champions were projecting their experience based on an equally limited group—cancer patients—across the wide realm of pain sufferers. "Arguments both pro and con are based on small segments of the pain populations with unique psychosocial and behavioral, as well as disease characteristics," he wrote.

In that same publication, a leading authority on substance abuse, Dr. Seedon R. Savage of Dartmouth Medical School, sounded another warning. Dr. Savage argued there was every reason to believe that the typical rate of substance abuse found in the general population—a range of 3 to 16 percent, with 10 percent the most referenced figure—might also hold true for pain patients put on strong narcotics for long periods. She noted that addiction risks for pain patients were likely to rise the longer they used drugs.

"It is tempting to dismiss all concerns regarding therapeutic opioids use as irrelevant," Savage wrote in 1996, adding:

That would clearly be a mistake. Many pain specialists who enthusiastically embraced the possibility of long-term opioid therapy for the treatment of chronic pain have been startled by the unanticipated consequences of such use which were not observed in previous experience with acute pain and cancer pain because the clinical variables in each of these settings differ significantly. Historical cautions regarding opioids use are not without basis.

Many years later Russell Portenoy would remember a trip around 1990 to the headquarters of Purdue Frederick, which was then located in Norwalk, Connecticut. Portenoy met with the company's top management team and scientists to argue that it was time for Purdue to start marketing a strong, long-acting narcotic like its morphine-based cancer drug, MS Contin, for chronic noncancer pain.

Portenoy recalled that his idea was not enthusiastically received. "I never heard back from them," he would say. "I just assumed that it was too hot, the connotation was too negative."

Such an idea, however, was already on Purdue's drawing board, and thanks in part to the momentum created by Portenoy's research, it soon emerged.

At the time of OxyContin's launching in 1996 it must have appeared to Purdue executives and their allies in the pain management movement that only vast opportunities beckoned. Medical and public awareness of untreated pain had been kindled, the perception of narcotics risk had been minimized, and regulatory initiatives had been slowed. The pendulum had dramatically swung. Quickly, sales of the new painkiller boomed, bringing record profits to Purdue and setting the small drugmaker on the path to realizing its dream of becoming a pharmaceutical powerhouse.

CHAPTER FOUR

MAGIC BULLETS

IN EARLY 1998, HERBERT Schaepe of the International Narcotics Control Board was scrolling through data in his office in the Austrian city of Vienna when he noticed something unusual. The statistics showed that on Tasmania, an island off the southern coast of Australia, commercial harvests of highly specialized breeds of opium poppy were rising. So were shipments from Tasmania to the United States of thebaine, the derivative of opium used to make oxycodone.

It is the job of the International Narcotics Control Board, or INCB, which is affiliated with the United Nations, to monitor such trends. The group acts as a worldwide narcotic watchdog, collecting data on illegal drug trafficking as well as the production of legal narcotics by pharmaceutical makers. It works closely with the U.S. Drug Enforcement Administration, which sets quotas on the amount of raw narcotics, like morphine, that can be imported into this country annually, and the volume of painkillers that drugmakers can produce. Both the INCB and the DEA have the same stated goal: to ensure that adequate narcotics supplies are available for medical needs while preventing their diversion into illegal activities such as the street sale of prescription drugs.

Schaepe soon learned from drug industry officials that the fast-growing sales of one painkiller, OxyContin, were driving the increasing demand for Tasmanian thebaine. But Schaepe was seeing only one sign of a far larger and more dramatic change then under way—the wholesale reshaping of a little-known but critical sector of the pharmaceutical industry.

For decades, drugmakers who sold narcotics had inhabited a quiet industry backwater content to make profits without drawing public attention to their products. It was a small, tightly knit industry. But some players in the field were big drugmakers and, in fact, household names. For instance, a division of Johnson & Johnson, the drug industry giant best known for baby powder and Band-Aids, was for many years one of only two companies permitted to import raw morphine into the United States; the other was the Mallinckrodt Corporation, a major producer of medical devices and hospital equipment. Meanwhile, other J&J units have long sold pain products. While the Duragesic patch, which is used to treat severe pain, is marketed by one J&J division, Janssen Pharmaceuticals, another division, Ortho-McNeil, sells Tylox, a general-use painkiller that contains a combination of oxycodone and acetaminophen. Until the mid-1990s, one of the world's biggest companies, DuPont, owned the Endo Company, the producer of Percodan and Percocet, both oxycodone-containing painkillers. In 2001, Abbott Laboratories, another drug industry powerhouse, acquired Knoll Laboratories, the maker of Vicodin, the popular prescription painkiller that is a combination of the narcotic hydrocodone and acetaminophen.

The pain management movement, along with cleansing the image of narcotics, had set off huge increases in the demand for such drugs. By the mid-1990s, narcotics producers were racing to supply those orders, and the events in Tasmania offered an extraordinary glimpse into one way they were trying to do so. There, researchers for J&J and another major drug company, Glaxo Wellcome of England, both had been quietly working on a remarkable project: the creation of specialized varieties of opium poppies to increase worldwide supplies of thebaine, oxycodone's starting material.

The companies, though competitors, were both trying to solve the same botanical problem. For decades the American pharmaceutical industry had relied on opium poppies grown in either India or Turkey as its prime source of morphine and other raw narcotics. The U.S. government, starting in the 1960s, had guaranteed the two countries a virtual monopoly on that market as an incentive to help stop the diversion of morphine into the black market, where it is converted into heroin. Under the initiative, which is known as the 80-20 Rule, India and Turkey became the designated suppliers of 80 percent of morphine and codeine destined for American drugmakers, with the remaining supplies coming from other countries.

But the policy had another consequence. Indian poppies, while producing high levels of morphine, yielded extremely small amounts of thebaine. This placed something of a natural cap on the amount of oxycodone available to narcotics producers. By the late 1980s, however, Tasmanian Alkaloids, a J&J unit, and Glaxo Wellcome both realized that pharmaceutical demand for thebaine was set to boom. And they were free to produce as much as they could because the 80-20 Rule that had given dominance to India and Turkey in morphine sales to American drug manufacturers didn't apply to thebaine.

As a result, the two pharmaceutical companies launched separate efforts on Tasmania to deal with the thebaine shortfall by producing new poppy varieties. The island was an ideal spot because its hot, sunny climate made it fertile ground for opium poppies and its surrounding waters served as a natural barrier against thieves.

Researchers for the companies tackled the thebaine problem using approaches similar to those of Gregor Mendel, the nineteenth-century botanist whose experiments with peas created the science of genetics. But unlike Mendel, they didn't have to wait for each successive generation of pea plant to pop out of the ground. Instead, high-speed laboratory techniques were used to crossbreed opium varieties and select out desirable qualities. By the mid-1990s both companies had succeeded in developing high-thebaine-yielding poppy strains. The new varieties soon bloomed in Tasmanian fields, their soft, pinkish-white flowers resplendent in the sunshine. Much of that harvest's bounty of thebaine was imported into the United States by the Noramco division of J&J, which then converted it into oxycodone for use in company products like Tylox or for sale to other narcotics producers. Before long, the big customer was Purdue.

Just around the time of Russell Portenoy's visit to Purdue, company researchers had already started working on a timed-release version of oxycodone. But the project initially hit stumbling blocks. The morphine in the company's timed-release MS Contin was contained within a waxy matrix that slowly dissolved. But oxycodone was a different chemical and the same slow-release technique apparently didn't work for it. So company scientists went back to the drawing board, eventually coming up with a new timed-release system for OxyContin that used a synthetic acrylic, rather than wax, as the basis of the tablet. The design provided a quick burst of oxycodone for pain relief as the pill's outer coating dissolved in the stomach. Then, as it moved from the stomach into the intestines, the acrylic tablet continued to release a steady supply of the drug over twelve hours.

OxyContin, like MS Contin before it, was essentially old wine in a new bottle, though an improved one from a medical perspective. The first painkiller sold in the United States that contained oxycodone, Percodan, which was a combination of the narcotic and aspirin, was introduced around 1950. It wasn't long, however, before oxycodone developed a reputation as a highly addictive narcotic attractive to drug abusers.

In 1963, California's attorney general, Stanley Mosk, blamed Percodan misuse for up to one-quarter of all drug addiction in that state, saying the company had marketed the drug too freely. A top Endo executive disputed the claim, maintaining that the painkiller possessed "relatively little or no addicting liability," the term used by abuse experts and pharmaceutical companies to describe a medication's attractiveness as a drug of abuse. However, officials of the Federal Bureau of Narcotics, the forerunner of today's DEA, came to a different conclusion. At the end of 1963 that agency ordered a nationwide tightening of prescribing controls on the drug.

"We're satisfied after a year's study that there has been an abuse of oral prescriptions as regards Percodan," one Bureau of Narcotics official said at the time. "We want to nip this in the bud and avert what might develop into a serious situation."

Later, a number of painkillers like Percocet that combined oxycodone with the aspirin substitute acetaminophen appeared. But unlike such combination products, OxyContin was pure oxycodone, or a single-entity drug, as such pharmaceuticals are known.

In the early 1990s, Purdue officials started submitting test data on OxyContin to the FDA as part of the lengthy process required of any pharmaceutical company that wants to get a new drug approved. As with any medication, patient trials of OxyContin served as the critical proving ground for the drug. Purdue studied OxyContin in various groups of patients, such as those who had cancer, osteoarthritis, or lower back pain . The drug's effect was also examined in people recovering from surgery. Since patient response to OxyContin alone would mean little by itself, the relative effectiveness of the drug was measured by giving other patients in the study groups pills other than OxyContin, such as an immediate-release form of pure oxycodone, a "combination" painkiller like Percocet, or a placebo like a sugar pill.

Purdue executives believed that their data showed that Oxy-Contin was not only more effective in killing pain than immediate-release forms of oxycodone but also posed fewer of the side effects traditionally associated with narcotics, such as nausea, dizziness, and constipation. As a result, they had high hopes that FDA officials would allow them to claim that Oxy-Contin was superior to competing painkillers that contained oxycodone.

FDA examiner Curtis Wright headed the agency's team that reviewed Purdue's data, and he was far less enthusiastic about what he saw. Wright dismissed Purdue's claim that OxyContin posed few side effects and concluded that its major benefit was that it needed to be taken only twice daily instead of six times a day, as was the case for shorter-acting drugs like Tylox.

"Care should be taken to limit competitive promotion," he wrote in a 1995 FDA report. "This product has been shown to be as good as current therapy, but has not been shown to have a significant advantage beyond a reduction in frequency of dosing."

To be sure, the advantage of a drug that has to be taken only twice daily wasn't insignificant for people enduring constant, severe pain. It allowed them to sleep through the night and avoid the discomfort during the day caused by waiting for doses of shorter-acting drugs to kick in. Doctors also like longer-lasting drugs; they believe that the fewer times patients have to take a dose, the less apt they are to miss one.

But in 1995 the trouble was that the FDA didn't require narcotics makers to run studies of how their painkillers might be abused in the real world. Nor did Purdue voluntarily undertake such tests. Company officials would later say there was no need to do so because they never intended challenging OxyContin's listing as a Schedule II narcotic, the category that identifies a prescription medication as having the greatest potential for abuse. However, executives of the drugmaker did receive something special from the FDA—a labeling claim so unique that no drug manufacturer had ever gotten a similar one. It implied that OxyContin, because it was a timed-release drug, posed a lower risk of abuse than other narcotic painkillers.

OxyContin would carry a warning on its package insert that was virtually similar in wording to the one that Purdue had used on MS Contin. Both products alerted doctors and users that breaking, chewing, or crushing a tablet could release a "potentially toxic" dose of its active narcotic. Such an acute overdose danger was particularly high for so-called opioid-naïve patients or those whose bodies hadn't as yet adapted to the physical effects of a strong narcotic like morphine or oxycodone.

OxyContin's label would also note that oxycodone-containing painkillers are "common targets for both drug abusers and drug addicts." But Purdue executives received permission from the FDA to imply that OxyContin had less appeal as a drug of abuse than competing narcotics because it was a timd-release product. Not only had no other manufacturer of a Schedule II narcotic ever got the go ahead from the FDA to make such a claim, but Purdue itself had not done so for MS Contin, even though it too was a timed-release medication.

Years later, a top company executive would say in a lawsuit deposition that FDA officials had suggested the unique labeling language and Curtis Wright, the FDA examiner, who would later go on to work for Purdue would support that version of events when questioned by plaintiffs' lawyers in 2003. But in a 1993 document submitted by Purdue to the FDA as part of OxyContin's approval process, officials of the drug company laid out what they saw as its potential advantages from a drug abuse perspective:

> A controlled-release formulation of oxycodone may have less abuse potential than drugs such as Percodan for several reasons. First, most illicit drug abusers prefer a drug that is rapidly acting. The controlled-release formulation will have a longer acting effect without producing an immediate euphoria. In addition, the tablet formulation of the controlled-release oxycodone will be more difficult to dissolve in a solution, hence not desired by the "street" addict, who prefers an injectable solution. Second, the controlled-release formulation of oxycodone will not be targeted for patients who might otherwise be

treated with codeine [a painkiller with less abuse potential than oxycodone] as has been the case [by some makers of oxycodone-containing drugs like Percodan] in the past. As previously stated, this controlled-release formulation of oxycodone will be useful in the treatment of patients with acute or chronic moderate to moderately-severe pain. In this regard, controlled-release oxycodone should be viewed by the prescribing physician as an alternative to morphine.

Purdue officials never conducted any of their own studies with drug abusers to determine their interest in OxyContin relative to other narcotics or to gauge the ease by which they could defeat its timed-release system. Instead, FDA and company officials apparently relied on limited research that supported the hypothesis that drug abusers appeared to prefer immediate-release narcotics to timed-release ones because the traditional painkillers offered a quicker buzz.

In one such survey, for example, Dr. Daniel Brookoff reported in a 1993 issue of the *Journal of Internal Medicine* that interviews with 130 hospital patients who had acknowledged abusing prescription narcotics found that 109 of them, or 85 percent, had tried to abuse controlled-release painkillers. Of that group, 65 patients, or 60 percent, reported that timed-release narcotics such as MS Contin were of "little or no use" to them and speculated that such painkillers would have low street value. As a result, Dr. Brookoff concluded, "These results suggest that controlled-release narcotic formulations may have a lower potential for abuse than do other narcotic medications. In situations where there is concern about potential abuse or diversion of prescribed narcotics, controlled-release preparations may be an appropriate alternative to high-peaking, rapid-onset opioid formulations."

The problem with Dr. Brookoff's study was that it, like similar studies, was based on an appealing hypothesis. Purdue officials would later say they did studies to support the theory but that theory would quickly collide with a far different reality when OxyContin began appearing on the streets of towns like Pennington Gap and started falling into the hands of teenagers such as Lindsay Myers. Nonetheless, FDA officials in December 1995 approved the sale of OxyContin with a label that read: "Delayed absorption, as provided by OxyContin tablets, is believed to reduce the abuse liability of a drug." It was a claim that soon became a cornerstone of the marketing of Oxy-Contin. And it was a decision that FDA officials would later come to regret.

Over the past hundred years, drug companies, scientists, and even the U.S. government have chased the dream of creating a "magic bullet," a drug as powerful in its painkilling effect as morphine but free of its pitfalls. In some ways the history of narcotics is a march of such substances, each one offered as a safer alternative to the addicting painkiller that preceded it.

Morphine, for instance, was initially thought to be less addictive than opium, and heroin was first marketed in 1898 as a morphine substitute safer than morphine. For a time some physicians even championed heroin as a cure for morphine addiction, but its extraordinary addictive powers soon became evident, and heroin's manufacture was banned in 1924. Then, in the early 1930s, another new narcotic, Dilaudid, generically known as hydromorphone, was introduced amid claims that it was a nonaddicting substitute for morphine. Not long afterward, its abuse was so widespread that Dilaudid was nicknamed "drugstore heroin."

It was also in the 1930s that the federal government launched its own effort to find a nonaddicting painkiller, a search that lasted four decades. Federal officials designated two prisons—one in Lexington, Kentucky, and the other in Fort Worth, Texas—as special facilities to house and rehabilitate drug addicts as well as to test the addictiveness of prospective painkillers on them. The Lexington facility, which was called the Farm, was the better known of the two prison-hospitals. Its test population was composed of prisoners who earned time off their sentences by volunteering to be subjects in drug trials. Civilian volunteers from outside the prison's walls were also used. Over the years at Lexington a number of compounds were tested, including one promising painkiller called dihydrodeoxymorphine-D, or desomorphine. Soon, however, its addicting nature was revealed. The tests at Lexington ended in the 1970s following revelations concerning earlier government-run experiments—the infamous Tuskegee studies in which four hundred black men infected with syphilis were allowed to go untreated for decades while scientists studied them.

Narcotics are by no means the only category of prescription drugs misused. There was an explosion of amphetamine abuse in the 1960s as pills known as "yellowjackets" and "black beauties" flooded the streets. The Valium-popping starlets of Jacquelin Susann's novel, *The Valley of the Dolls*, symbolized American society's vast appetite for tranquilizers in the 1970s. Not long afterward, the abuse of Quaaludes, a sedative, became commonplace.

But while prescription-drug abusers may differ in their pharmaceutical choices, the dynamic of abuse shares a common theme: whatever a manufacturer's claims about a drug's "abuse liability," both hard-core drug addicts and recreational users will quickly find ways to make a drug their own.

In the late 1960s, for instance, Sterling Drug Inc. announced that it had synthesized a new drug called pentazocine that had painkilling properties similar to those of morphine but not its addiction dangers. The company said its findings were based on testing the drug, which it sold as Talwin, on thousands of people, including inmates at the Lexington prison facility.

However, heroin users, facing shortages of that substance, soon discovered a way to get a heroin-like high from Talwin. No one claimed credit for the achievement, but it required some ingenuity; when Talwin was dissolved together with a widely available antihistamine, the resulting brew created an injectable speedball that served as a heroin substitute. On the street the mixture became known as "T's and Blues."

By the mid-1970s the abuse of Talwin had become so severe that Sterling was forced to reformulate the drug. The company did so by adding a substance called naloxone to the painkiller. Naloxone is derived from the opium poppy but acts as a narcotic blocker that prevents morphine and similar substances from producing a high in a user's brain. Naloxone, which is also known as Narcan, is frequently used in hospital emergency rooms; its administration quickly brings down an overdose victim. An addict shooting up the reformulated version of Talwin, which was sold as Talwin NX, risked the same reaction. Naloxone, however, didn't interfere with the reformulated drug's painkilling properties because when Talwin NX was taken orally as intended, the naloxone in it was neutralized in the stomach. Soon after the appearance of Talwin NX in the early 1980s, the drug's abuse began to decline.

Twenty years later, many of those who would abuse or experiment with OxyContin weren't hard-core drug addicts but teenagers and young people such as Lindsay Myers looking for a new thrill. And for kids like Lindsay, unlike Talwin abusers a decade earlier, defeating OxyContin's timed-release system required little ingenuity; on the contrary, it was child's play.

Of the drug abuse counselors working in and around Lee County, it was probably Larry Lavender who noticed Oxy-Contin first. Lavender, like Sister Beth Davies, was used to working with people who were abusing or were addicted to painkillers or tranquilizers. But in 1999 a local physician, Dr. Richard Norton, started sending some of his pain patients to the addiction counselor so he could try to determine whether they were suitable candidates for treatment with a powerful narcotic like OxyContin.

Years later, Lavender, a stocky man who wore a short brown ponytail and a small gold hoop earring, would remember one of Norton's patients in particular. At the time, Lavender was practicing in the town of Big Stone Gap, about twenty miles northeast of Pennington Gap. As he sat in Lavender's office the man explained how OxyContin was working wonders for his lower back pain and how important it was for Norton to keep him on it. But to Lavender's trained eye, the man was exhibiting all the classic signs of drug-abusing behavior. He explained, for instance, that he had somehow misplaced his vial of OxyContins and needed a new prescription for the painkiller right away. It also turned out that he had just lost his job and that his wife had walked out on him, taking their children. However, none of that seemed to matter more to the man than getting the drug.

In making his assessment, Lavender had the advantage of personal experience. The son of an addict, he had started messing with drugs at age thirteen and was shooting heroin by high school. It was a habit that got him kicked out of the Air Force and had landed him in jail. On a night in 1985, Lavender found himself standing at the edge of Baltimore's inner harbor with nothing on but a pair of dirty blue jeans, holding a gun in his hand. He planned to kill himself, but for a reason he never fully understood, he decided to make a phone call. After going through treatment, he started a new life as a substance abuse counselor, eventually moving to southwestern Virginia with his wife and children.

As he started seeing more of Dr. Norton's patients, Lavender's concerns grew. He knew that some of them had abused other narcotics in the past and that others had quickly become addicted to OxyContin. In referring patients to Lavender, Norton was taking a sensible precaution. But Lavender would later say that Norton never followed his advice about taking some patients off the drug.

Because OxyContin was such a new drug at the time, Lavender decided in late 1999 to call Greg Stewart, a pharmacist in Pennington Gap, to get more information about it. Stewart told him that he was worried about Norton's prescribing because many of the physician's patients, including those with past drug problems, had started to come to his pharmacy to have their OxyContin prescriptions filled. Other of Norton's patients weren't even local. Instead, Stewart told Lavender, they were coming to see the physician from towns in Kentucky and Tennessee.

Stewart later recalled how he had eventually called Norton to discuss his prescribing. The physician's response was brief; Norton told the pharmacist: "I don't need a dissertation about addiction, Greg."

When the sale of OxyContin began in 1996, Purdue executives could hardly have foreseen the widespread abuse of the drug that would quickly unfold. The company's timed-release morphine painkiller, MS Contin, already had been used for more than a decade in places such as the controlled confines of cancer wards where there was little to indicate that it was being misused. Instead, Purdue had another type of problem with MS Contin that it hoped to cure with OxyContin. Since its launch in 1984, cancer specialists had embraced MS Contin as the gold standard for treatment of the disease's most severe pain. And a decade later, it held a commanding 80 percent share of that market; sales of the drug in 1995 reached about $110 million, or some 25 percent of Purdue's total income.

The drug had few competitors, such as J&J's pain patch, Duragesic. But the patent on MS Contin, Purdue's flagship product, was soon set to expire, a development that would open the door for generic drug producers to market cheaper, knockoff versions of MS Contin.

Purdue, like any other drug company, wasn't about to wait for generic producers to take away its business. It had a strategy ready: to convince cancer specialists to switch from MS Contin to OxyContin, a drug with a fresh patent.

Purdue officials also saw OxyContin as a way not only to hold but to expand their cancer treatment franchise. Doctors reserved morphine-based drugs like MS Contin for use against cancer's most severe pain. For stages of the disease when its pain was moderate, they had traditionally relied on combination medications like Percocet or Vicodin. But executives believed that OxyContin could also grab a large share of the moderate cancer pain market away from such drugs. Then, cancer specialists could keep using the new painkiller throughout the course of the disease, increasing dosages as a patient's pain increased.

OxyContin's first two years on the market were relatively

low-key as Purdue worked to build up a network to distribute, promote, and sell the new drug. In 1996, Purdue forged a deal with Abbott Laboratories under which the larger pharmaceutical company's sales force would promote OxyContin to hospitals.

But from the beginning, Purdue executives had far more ambitious visions for their new painkiller. They planned to make it among the first pure and powerful pain medications mass-marketed for a wide range of conditions unrelated to cancer—like lower back pain, arthritis, surgical pain, fibromyalgia, dental surgery pain, and pain resulting from broken bones, sports injuries, and trauma.

"In 1997, OxyContin will be launched into the non-malignant market," one company budget document from 1996 stated. "The most common diagnoses for non-malignant pain are back pain, osteoarthritis, injury, and trauma pain. The major competitors for these diagnoses will be oxycodone and hydrocodone combination products, as well as Ultram. Oxy-Contin will be positioned as providing the equivalent efficacy and safety of combination opioids, with the benefit of" twice-daily dosing.

The timing of OxyContin's launch couldn't have been better. By now the awareness of both patients and doctors about the inadequate treatment of pain had been heightened. Pain as a medical science was coming into its own and, in a few short years, doctors and nurses in every hospital in the United States would be required to routinely monitor patient pain and treat it. In addition, oxycodone didn't have the same stigma as morphine, which patients often associated with terminal disease.

Even before OxyContin's formal approval in late 1995, company marketing strategists were devising plans to hammer home a message that the company would constantly repeat: pain was America's silent epidemic and untold millions of patients were suffering unnecessarily because of its undertreatment.

"In an effort to create a 'media hook' that would coincide with the launch of OxyContin, a consumer survey conducted by a company such as The Gallop [sic] Poll is being proposed," one Purdue executive wrote earlier that year. "This survey would focus on the prevalence and problems of chronic pain, both malignant and non-malignant. The release of the results of such a survey would be publicized along with the recent FDA approval of a new controlled-release Oxycodone preparation; OxyContin. This is a classic problem/solution strategy to create a need for the launch of a product such as OxyContin."

It's not clear whether such a survey was conducted at that time. But a subsequent one in 2000 underwritten by Purdue found the problem of pain to be of such staggering proportion that it seemed a miracle that most Americans ever got out of bed. Its key "finding": at least one family member in 44 million households nationwide—or nearly one-half of the homes in the United States—suffered from chronic pain.

"Why does this suffering continue?" one publicity release issued around that time by a public relations firm working for

Purdue asked rhetorically. "Underuse of opioids (narcotics), such as morphine and codeine, is one reason."

To reach patients, the drug company expanded an existing public relations operation called Partners Against Pain, which operated an Internet site that provided pain sufferers with, among other things, referrals to doctors. Soon pamphlets and videotapes produced by Purdue that encouraged patients to talk with their physicians about pain began to appear in doctors' waiting rooms.

Still, the ultimate audience that Purdue had to win over was the people holding the prescribing pens—doctors. So not long after OxyContin's launch, Purdue began paying the travel and hotel costs of doctors to attend three-day seminars on pain management in resort locations like Arizona, California, and Florida. The theme of those meetings was pain's widespread "undertreatment" and the need for doctors to address the problem by more aggressively prescribing long-acting narcotics like OxyContin.

In time, an estimated two thousand to three thousand doctors would attend those weekend meetings. Purdue also used the events to recruit hundreds of doctors for its speakers bureau, a roster of physicians whom pharmaceutical companies typically pay to give talks. Some of Purdue's speakers, like Dr. Susan Bertrand of the Appalachian Pain Foundation, received honorariums of about $500 per talk; better-known pain experts earned upwards of $3,000. These medical foot soldiers covered a wide terrain, speaking at every possible venue, including hospitals, meetings of local medical societies, and get-togethers or continuing educational programs for nurses, pharmacists, and others in the medical field. When marketing MS Contin, Purdue had positioned itself as a pain management "educator" and had already earned a position of respect among cancer specialists and pain experts.

But this time, in 1996, its prime audience wasn't specialists. Instead, Purdue took its advocacy of powerful narcotics straight into medicine's heartland, the offices of family doctors, general practitioners, and other physicians who lacked skills in pain management and training in how to recognize patients prone to prescription drug abuse. By Purdue's own estimate, the company sponsored thousands of such talks in the years following the new painkiller's launch. Officials of the drugmaker always insisted when asked by reporters that the talks were generic in nature, intended only to raise medical awareness about the inadequacy of pain treatment rather than to market OxyContin. But any program promoting the use of long-acting narcotics also promoted OxyContin. The reason: the number of competing products could be counted on a few fingers.

Years later, Purdue's internal documents—disclosed as part of an investigation by Florida state officials into the drug's marketing—made clear that company executives viewed any discussion of pain management and long-acting narcotics as beneficial to its business interests. The company's 1998 budget lists several "communication objectives," including a push "to convince health care professionals (physicians, nurses, pharmacists, and managed care professionals) to aggressively treat both non-cancer pain and cancer pain. The positive use of opioids, and OxyContin tablets in particular, will be emphasized."

The same document also makes it clear that Purdue's marketing strategy went far beyond trying to convince doctors to use OxyContin only after other less powerful painkillers had failed to work. Instead, the company wanted to persuade physicians to prescribe its new narotic for some patients even before trying these other drugs, including one called Ultram, a nonnarcotic generically known as tramadol, which is classified as having a far lower potential for abuse than OxyContin.

In the company's 1998 budget plan, which was written the previous year, Purdue executives described that goal:

> To convince MDs to prescribe, as well as RNs and appropriate pharmacists to recommend, OxyContin Tablets for both opioid-naïve or opioid-exposed patients with moderate-to-severe pain lasting more than a few days instead of combination opioids and Ultram and, through proper dosing and [dosage adjustment], eliminate or delay the need for other long-acting opioids.

For Purdue, the selling of OxyContin was the most ambitious undertaking in company history. By 1998 the company's sales force would stand at about 625 people, nearly twice its level prior to OxyContin's introduction. And about 70 percent of those reps were detailed to promoting the company's new painkiller.

Purdue had little trouble recruiting sales reps because its sales-based bonus system was considered to be among the most lucrative in the pharmaceutical industry. Before long, some of those selling OxyContin were earning annual bonuses of $100,000 or more.

Each new salesman or saleswoman hired by Purdue received three weeks of training with four days specifically devoted to MS Contin and OxyContin. The programs, which were conducted at the company's headquarters, included presentations on the history of pain care, its science, and the company's mission to better it. They were also schooled in the basics of pain medicine from the perspective of narcotics advocates. During such training sessions, sales reps were quizzed on lessons learned, including one question concerning the risk of iatrogenic addiction posed by narcotics to pain patients. The correct answer was "less than one percent."

Following training, each sales rep then went out into the field to work a specific geographic territory under the supervision of a district area manager. Purdue equipped its reps with the most modern pharmaceutical marketing tools available. The company, like other drugmakers, utilized the services of a little-known Philadelphia-area firm called IMS Health, which operates a vast data-mining network that provides pharmaceutical producers exquisitely detailed looks at which medications physicians prescribe, and how frequently they do so. To do that, IMS routinely collects computer data showing recently filled prescriptions from more than 50 percent of the pharmacies in the United States and, by using sophisticated projections, can tell a drugmaker not only how many times a specific physician has prescribed its products, but also the dosage strengths ordered. While patient names on prescriptions are stripped out for confidentiality reasons, drugmakers can also learn what type of insurance—private or taxpayer funded—is used to pay for their products.

By contrast, DEA and state officials, who also attempt to track narcotics use, stumble around in the dark. The data available to them show only shipments to a pharmacy of classes of substances—all oxycodone-containing painkillers, for example—rather than specific brands. And only states with prescription monitoring had anything even remotely comparable to IMS data that would also allow them to determine quickly which doctors were using what drugs.

With IMS data, Purdue reps knew not only how much Oxy-Contin a doctor was prescribing but also how many prescriptions he or she was writing for competing painkillers, allowing them to better tailor their sales pitches. The reps had access to an internal company Internet site that updated IMS data as soon as new statistics were available. Purdue marketing officials also massaged the data into reports that were then placed on the same Internet site with names like Outlet Zip Report, Core Coverage Report, and Combo Opportunity Report. The latter was a reference to doctors who were good sales targets because they were already prescribing high volumes of combination drugs like the painkillers Percocet and Vicodin. In Purdue's marketing lingo, doctors were ranked, according to their prescribing volume, as "decibels," with a decibel 10 the highest.

Doctors who were classified as decibels 8 through 10 were considered prime opportunities.

In making their pitches, Purdue reps pointed to OxyContin's longer-lasting action and its purity as advantages over traditional painkillers. But company reps continued to face a major hurdle: convincing doctors, still leery of the specter of narcotics abuse and addiction, that a powerful painkiller like OxyContin was safe. In fact, surveys of doctors commissioned by Purdue just before and after OxyContin's launch indicated that the drug might be doomed to be a niche product. Doctors might prescribe OxyContin for severe pain, the studies found, but few were interested in using it to treat those in moderate pain, a far bigger market, because they considered it too strong or too much of an abuse risk. In that regard, the FDA had given Purdue a powerful marketing weapon.

In November 1996, about a year after OxyContin's approval by the agency, every Purdue sales rep received a training memo on the subject of planning an effective presentation to doctors about OxyContin. It was entitled "If I Only Had a Brain . . ." The introduction to the memo read:

> In *The Wizard of Oz*, Dorothy had a clear-cut objective. She knew exactly what she wanted—to get back home to Kansas. Who could help her? Only one person could give her what she wanted: The Wizard. According to the munchkins, the Right Approach (how to accomplish this task) was to take the Yellow Brick Road. The attention-grabber was Dorothy's painting-the-picture of her Auntie

Em. Turns out that Dorothy knew that the guard also had an Auntie Em. That got them inside. Toto eventually grabbed the Wizard's attention by pulling down his curtain. Then Dorothy knew she had to "ask" for his attention.

As doctors' scheduling demands are getting tighter, you need to more effectively plan your presentations.

The memo went on to lay out a general sales strategy for reps to use in meetings with doctors. It suggested, among other things, that they point to the FDA-approved labeling language for OxyContin to address physician concern about the drug's addictive potential:

Know your listener and his/her needs/wants: Gather facts about your customer prior to your call. Firing at a target in the dark is not very promising. As you prepare to fire your "message," you need to know where to aim and what you want to hit! "The physician wants pain relief for these patients without addicting them to an opioid."

Have a Well-formulated Approach: A single thought or sentence that will best lead you to your objective. "According to the FDA, stated in the OxyContin package insert, 'Drug addiction is characterized with the procurement, hoarding and abuse of drugs for non-medicinal purposes.' 'Delayed absorption, as provided by OxyContin tablets, is believed to reduce the abuse liability of a drug.'"

The memo, which contained other sales tips, closed on an up-beat note also drawn from *The Wizard of Oz*. It reminded each sales rep that "A pot of gold awaits you 'Over the Rainbow'!"

Some Purdue reps made that message of implied safety a key component of their efforts to convince doctors to prescribe OxyContin and encourage pharmacists to stock it in drugstores. The sales pitch was typically aimed against short-acting drugs like Percocet, Lortab, and Vicodin that were known targets for abusers.

"They were going around to doctors promoting that this was the answer to all abuse," an owner of a drugstore in southern Indiana, John Craig, would later tell the *New York Times*. A Purdue sales rep, Craig recalled, kept telling him that OxyContin "could not be crushed. It could not be injected."

One former Purdue district sales manager, William Gergely, told an investigator in the Florida attorney general's office that top company marketing and sales executives had described OxyContin to him and sales officials as "non-habit forming." Greg Stewart, the druggist in downtown Pennington Gap, later recalled how a Purdue saleswoman had walked into his pharmacy to offer him similar assurances about OxyContin long before Dr. Richard Norton started writing prescriptions for it.

"She said drug abusers won't be interested in it," Stewart remembered.

Two years later that claim would be hard to make in places like Lee County. "Nearly every person in my county is now familiar with the slang name Oxys," the county's sheriff, Gary

Parsons, wrote in a letter in November 2000. "I would say that easily as much as 70 percent of our theft crimes in this county are tied directly to OxyContin. Young people's lives are being destroyed every day by these pills. We are in desperate need in Southwest Virginia for some type of help in dealing with this epidemic of drug abuse."

Police officials like Sheriff Parsons weren't the only people working overtime. Half a world away, opium farmers in Tasmania were tilling the soil to prepare it for more poppy plantings. And closer to Lee County, a Purdue plant in New Jersey that made OxyContin was operating at a breakneck pace, running double shifts to feed a booming demand.

CHICKEN
AND
BISCUITS

ART VAN ZEE FELT HE had an inordinate amount of patience, but by the late fall of 2000 he could sense it slipping away. OxyContin's abuse was now carving into the life of Lee County in ways he hadn't anticipated. He learned from child welfare investigators, for instance, that the number of children in foster care had doubled during the time OxyContin had taken hold in the area, as children went neglected by a drug-obsessed parent. Meanwhile, the region's few drug treatment centers were being overrun. One methadone clinic, prior to its opening in early 2000, had estimated that it would treat about 15 opiate addicts during its first year of operation. Six months later, more than 250 people a day were seeking treatment, the vast majority hooked on Oxys.

From Van Zee's perspective, the efforts that Purdue was making to contain the problem, like the seminars sponsored by the Appalachian Pain Foundation, weren't doing enough. So he decided the time had come for him to step in and play a bigger role. He started reading articles in medical journals about prescription drug abuse; he also called experts in the field for their suggestions and advice. In the process he learned about Talwin, and how Sterling Drug had reformulated it with naloxone to reduce its abuse.

Van Zee was also swapping friendly e-mails with a Purdue medical official, Dr. Daniel Spyker, in which they discussed educational programs that the company might sponsor for area teenagers about prescription drug abuse. But by November of 2000 the tone of Van Zee's e-mails to Purdue also conveyed a mounting sense of urgency.

"I would suggest that Purdue needs to aggressively and seriously approach this problem," he wrote to Spyker. "Most important I think is that Purdue work toward reformulating OxyContin so that it is combined with naloxone—like what was done with the Talwin/NX situation. . . . Also important I think is that Purdue stop aggressive marketing of OxyContin in the treatment of chronic non-malignant pain. The real life experience for the proliferation of OxyContin in the treatment of chronic non-malignant pain in this and several other regions in the country has proved to be a medical, social, legal and societal catastrophe."

Van Zee also began planning a meeting of area doctors that he hoped would serve as a counterpoint to the one held by the

Appalachian Pain Foundation. Van Zee wanted his meeting to focus on prescription drug abuse and help area doctors and abuse counselors deal with the onslaught of OxyContin-addicted patients they were seeing.

In October 2000 he found two drug abuse treatment experts from Yale University to speak at the event: Dr. David Fiellin and Dr. Richard Schottenfeld. Van Zee made the rounds of local health care organizations to raise money to cover the meeting's costs and the professors' traveling expenses.

Sue Ella watched her husband's sudden burst of energy with hidden pleasure. For a time that fall she had worried that Van Zee might be sinking into a depression; he seemed so intent on spending hours by himself in his basement office. But now he had emerged with a sudden vigor. Sue Ella had long taken pride in her role as the family's resident activist, but if Art wanted to share that title, it was perfectly fine with her.

At the same time, Purdue executives were growing more aware of Art Van Zee. Soon after agreeing to speak at the Lee County gathering, Dr. Fiellin, one of the Yale experts, had contacted the drugmaker for information about the painkiller's abuse and his call was routed to David Haddox, the company's chief firefighter on the issue. The Purdue executive told Fiellin that he questioned the research methods that Van Zee and others in Lee County were using to estimate the problem's scope. If there was an "epidemic," Fiellin would later recall Haddox saying, it had to do with pain's inadequate treatment, not OxyContin's abuse.

Nonetheless, Van Zee was notified by Purdue in November

that Haddox planned to pass through southwestern Virginia and wanted to meet him for dinner. On the appointed day, Van Zee and Larry Lavender made the short drive to the town of Norton, where Van Zee had agreed to meet Haddox at a Holiday Inn.

Van Zee and Lavender were already at the Holiday Inn when Haddox arrived. The Purdue doctor apologized for being late; he had just come from a community meeting in a North Carolina town that was also dealing with OxyContin.

In the previous few months, Purdue's efforts to deal with the problems engulfing its painkiller had intensified. In September, for example, company officials flew to Maine for a meeting with the U.S. attorney Jay P. McCloskey, the prosecutor who had alerted state doctors earlier in 2000 about the drug's abuse. McCloskey told Purdue executives that given the painkiller's unfolding problems, he wanted them to end the weekend retreats they had been holding for doctors. Purdue executives agreed to do so and also started to put into place a plan aimed at combating the drug's misuse in Maine. It included expanded educational programs for doctors and pharmacists as well as the distribution of specially treated prescription pads that couldn't be duplicated in copying machines or easily forged, techniques used to create phony prescriptions. That same month the drug company brought twenty of its top consultants together for a meeting at an Atlanta hotel to discuss strategies to reduce the painkiller's growing diversion and abuse.

As they dined with Haddox on that November evening,

both Van Zee and Lavender were impressed with the company physician's extensive knowledge about drug abuse and addiction. He responded sympathetically when Lavender told him a story about one of his patients, a thirteen-year-old girl, who was shooting up OxyContin intravenously.

Van Zee had spent days preparing for this meeting with Haddox. Over coffee, Van Zee again raised his concerns that Purdue's broad marketing of OxyContin for various types of pain had helped fuel the outbreak by making the drug too easy to get. He then reached into his inside jacket pocket and pulled out a sheet of paper that he handed to Haddox. It was a list of actions that he wanted Purdue to take. It read:

1. Send a letter—red lettered—"ALERT"—to all physicians and mid-level practitioners calling attention to the fact that in some regions of the country there has been recognized large scale abuse of OxyContin (used IV or snorted) leading to opioid dependence with the associated medical, personal, and social consequences usually seen with opioid addiction;

2. Send an even more extensive ALERT notice to all physicians practicing in pain management positions or specialties;

3. Stop marketing OxyContin for use in chronic non-malignant pain by stopping all advertisements that promote its use in this situation—i.e., chronic, non-malignant pain;

4. Revise Purdue Pharma's web site to reflect that there has been reported in some regions in the country extensive abuse of OxyContin, and give a detailed picture;

5. Stop sponsorship of pain management seminars around the country that promote heavily the use of opioids for chronic non-malignant pain;

6. Examine carefully the data that Purdue has concerning its sales of OxyContin in those regions of the country that we know have extensive abuse—specifically southwest Virginia; the Cincinnati, Ohio, area; the Altoona, Pennsylvania, area; and Maine.

Do these particular areas have a significantly higher prescribing pattern for physicians for OxyContin—*i.e.*, in grams per 100,000 population area—are these areas where abuse is heavily seen, areas where there has also been much more frequent prescribing? etc.

Are these areas Purdue Pharma has chosen to market more heavily to physicians, etc. the use of OxyContin? What other factors can we identify that would explain this kind of regional diversity in the abuse of the drug?

8. Replace OxyContin with Oxy/Nx— oxycodone/naloxone, which would presumably cut down substantially on the amount of abuse of the drug.

Art Van Zee, M.D.

In typing out his wish list, Van Zee had inadvertently misnumbered it, going straight from number six to eight without stopping at seven. After glancing at the document, David Haddox assured Van Zee and Lavender that he would deliver it to Purdue executives at the company's headquarters. Then the three men wished each other good night. A few days later, Van Zee sent a follow-up letter to Haddox thanking him for his time and again suggesting that Purdue consider funding educational programs about drug abuse in southwestern Virginia schools. He also wrote a note to Dr. Daniel Spyker, the other Purdue executive with whom he had been corresponding. It read:

> Larry and I appreciated meeting with David Haddox the other night. I appreciate very much David's time and interest in these issues of mutual concern. David had asked for some of my practical suggestions and I did give him a list written out on 11/20/00. Some of these may seem harsh and unrealistic. However, I don't think anyone ever would have imagined the scope and magnitude of abuse of OxyContin that is appearing in regions around the country. My fear is that these are sentinel areas, just as San Francisco and New York were in the early years of HIV [the virus that causes AIDs]. I don't think any of us understand all the reasons why this is occurring. Therefore, until this is better understood and come to terms with, I do suggest these measures to stop promoting OxyContin for use in chronic non-malignant pain. I would think, until things are better understood as to what is going on, that this would be in the best interest of public health and Purdue.

Around the same time, Vince Stravino ran into Van Zee and asked him about how the meeting with Haddox had gone. Van

Zee said he was heartened because the Purdue executive seemed to have taken the situation so seriously.

"I think it's going to help," Van Zee said.

About ten days after Van Zee's dinner with Haddox, the Yale University drug abuse experts, David Fiellin and Richard Schottenfeld, arrived in Lee County. Before the meeting, Sister Beth Davies and Sister Elizabeth Vines gave them a tour of the area, driving past coal camps and pointing out houses where OxyContin dealers were operating. As he rode around southwestern Virginia, Fiellin was struck by something that had caught the attention of Art Van Zee three decades earlier: there still were hardly any medical services in the area. To find a pain specialist or a drug treatment program, Fiellin realized, people had to travel for hours.

Late that afternoon they arrived at a building that housed the community center in the tiny town of St. Paul, Virginia, about fifty miles east of Pennington Gap. Inside, a buffet-style dinner—platters of chicken and biscuits and bowls of salad—was laid out on tables for those attending the meeting. About 150 people soon made their way into the hall, many of them doctors who had come to Appalachia, like Vince Stravino, as Public Health Service physicians to pay back government loans.

Few of those attending the meeting had any experience with opiate addiction. Heroin had never been a substantial part of the drug scene in Appalachia; places like Lee County were just too far away from big cities that were the hubs of heroin dealing or even the interstate highways that served as trafficking routes. Now a legal drug, OxyContin, which was almost a match for heroin in its addictive power, had moved in. Experts don't know precisely why some people get addicted to a drug and others don't, but they suspect that a constellation of genetic, neurobiological, and social factors play a role. So the two Yale professors began the meeting by trying to convey a basic sense of the addiction process and the different ways to treat it.

Narcotics advocates like Russell Portenoy had long sought to reeducate doctors about the distinctions between physical and psychological dependency, but some drug abuse specialists did not believe that the line was always so clear. David Fiellin told the group gathered in St. Paul that the intense physical reaction and psychological stress caused by the sudden withdrawal of a narcotic played a role in the addiction syndrome. Put another way, for people like Lindsay Myers, the intense fear of going through the agony of withdrawal was one reason they stayed hooked. Fiellin explained that staying straight was a long and difficult road that many former addicts and drug abusers had to negotiate for the rest of their lives. While both he and Schottenfeld believed that OxyContin was an extremely useful medication, Fiellin remarked that Lee County wasn't the best setting for its use because the area clearly didn't have the resources to deal with the calamities resulting from the medication's misuse. As an alternative, he and Schottenfeld suggested

that local physicians prescribe other drugs to patients with severe pain, such as MS Contin, the Duragesic patch, or
methadone.

Toward the meeting's end, one man in the audience rose up
and sharply challenged both Van Zee and Richard Schottenfeld,
asking them whether they thought the problem of opioid abuse
would disappear if OxyContin was no longer prescribed. Van
Zee didn't answer the question directly but said he believed that
drug abuse incidents would decline if fewer OxyContin prescriptions were written. At the meeting's end, David Fiellin
learned the questioner's identity: he was a local sales rep for
Purdue.

In early December 2000, about a week after the meeting in St.
Paul, Art Van Zee again sat in his basement office, writing another letter. This one wasn't going to Purdue. A few days earlier Van Zee had called the headquarters of the FDA in
Rockville, Maryland, and been put in contact with Dr. Deborah
Leiderman, an official on the agency's controlled substances
staff. He had described to her the scope and nature of the Oxy-
Contin problem in southwestern Virginia and was now following up that conversation with a letter, one that he copied to
an official at the National Institute on Drug Abuse, another federal agency. In his letter to Dr. Leiderman, Van Zee described
the outbreaks of OxyContin abuse in Lee County and other
places, adding:

This is a problem that is not being written about in the medical literature. The experts in the pain management community promote the use of opioids for chronic non-malignant pain and Purdue Pharma has marketed aggressively for the use of opioids in chronic non-malignant pain. The real life experience for the liberal use of opioids has proven to be a medical and social disaster for our region, and as I fear, may be a glimpse of what will happen nationally over the next few years.

I would request that your office look into this further if at all possible. I could not over-state the major consequences this problem has had for our area. I have talked with Dr. Dan Spyker, senior medical director at Purdue Pharma. They are well aware of this problem. Among other things, I had suggested that a WARNING or URGENT NOTICE type of letter be sent to all physicians in the U.S. explaining that—at least in certain regions of the country—the OxyContin has been abused— snorted and injected—so as to lead to opioid dependence—and that all prescribing physicians need to be aware of this potential.

As he sealed the letter, Van Zee could sense that he was about to cross over a line he had never expected to reach.

If Art Van Zee's patience had run out, the same could be said about Jane Myers, who felt like she had come to the breaking point where Lindsay was concerned. In November 2000, right around the time that Van Zee was meeting with Purdue's David

Haddox, Jane had decided to go through Lindsay's bag again. Some of Lindsay's teachers had started calling the house asking about notes that Lindsay had brought in bearing Jane's signature. The notes asked Lindsay's teachers to excuse her from school for up to two weeks in some cases. They were clearly forgeries, but Jane decided to cover for Lindsay until she could get things sorted out.

Now, in going through Lindsay's purse, Jane was relieved to find only a roll of breath mints. She took one for herself. When she did, a pill fell out of the roll. In a fury she went storming back toward Lindsay's bedroom, holding the pill and the bag in her outstretched arm.

Lindsay saw her coming and waited until her mother's arm was in the room before pushing the door shut. Jane screamed out and there was a tug-of-war as Lindsay pressed on the door and Jane tried to free her arm. After a while they both started crying. Lindsay admitted the pill was a Percocet. She told her mother she was taking them to help wean herself off Oxy-Contin. Once again, Jane wanted to believe her and so she let it go.

The approach of Christmas presented a new concern. Jane's mother always gave generous holiday checks to Lindsay and the other grandchildren. But Jane decided that this year Lindsay wasn't going to get hers, so she couldn't spend it on drugs. She thought she could make it up to Lindsay by putting plenty of other presents out for her under the family's tree. One contained an expensive belt she thought Lindsay would love. But on Christmas morning, Lindsay's interest in her pile of beautifully wrapped packages perked up only when she heard a cousin thank their grandmother for his check.

"Mom, where is the money that Nana gave me?" she demanded to know. "Where is my envelope?"

"I'm taking care of it," Jane told her.

Lindsay glared at her mother before leaving the room. She was desperate for that check. Ray had broken his hip in early 2000 when he had smashed up an ATV and a doctor had put him on OxyContin. His prescriptions had been one source of the drug for them, but now Ray's prescription had been cut off and Lindsay had run out of money. It was becoming a daily struggle to scrape together enough to score something, even a Percocet. Things got so bad that one day Lindsay drove out on Skaggs Hill Road and crushed up a few Tylenols to snort, just to feel something in her nose.

Lindsay and Ray needed to find a doctor who was still freely writing prescriptions for Oxys, but given the law enforcement crackdown, it was getting harder to do that. Then, just after Christmas, Ray heard from friends about a doctor named Ali Sawaf in nearby Harlan, Kentucky. The word on the street was that Sawaf would write scripts for any drug a "patient" wanted.

When Lindsay and Ray arrived at Sawaf's office, about thirty people were squeezed into a tiny, dirty waiting room. To Lindsay, many of them looked strung out. She and Ray waited for an hour before his name was called. They had decided that he would be the patient because he had been prescribed Oxys for his hip. Lindsay watched Ray as he disappeared behind a door into the doctor's examining room. He emerged a few minutes later, smiling. When they got back into Lindsay's Jeep, she saw he had a prescription for sixty Oxy 40s and another one for sixty Xanax.

"What did he say?" Lindsay asked.

"He asked me what I wanted," he replied.

Lindsay and Ray first tried to get the Oxy prescription filled at the Rite-Aid pharmacy in Pennington Gap, but Sawaf's reputation for running a pill mill wasn't known only on the street. By now most area pharmacies were refusing to fill his prescriptions. Even Art Van Zee had heard about Sawaf. One of his patients called to say that dozens of teenagers in her town were walking around with OxyContin prescriptions they had gotten from the Harlan doctor. Van Zee and Larry Lavender toyed with the idea of conducting a sting operation in which they'd pose as patients and get Sawaf to write them prescriptions for Oxys, which they would then bring to the police. Van Zee had gone as far as making an appointment. But when he and Lavender mentioned their plans to Sue Ella, she told them not to get involved. "You'll probably screw up a really good DEA investigation," she said.

It took Lindsay and Ray two hours of driving around to get Sawaf's prescription filled. In a few weeks, the Oxys were gone, and by that time so was Sawaf. The Harlan physician had gotten busted for illegally prescribing OxyContin and other drugs. Once again, Lindsay and Ray were barely hanging on.

Then, one January morning, as Jane Myers was showering,

the bathroom door suddenly opened and Lindsay stuck her head in.

"Mom, I'm going out with Ray," her daughter announced.

Jane decided otherwise.

"You are absolutely not going out," she told her.

Lindsay let out a defiant grunt, picked up a phone, and began dialing. She shouted into the receiver so that her mother, who was still in the shower, could hear her.

"Ray," she yelled. "You come up here right now and get me."

Jane shut off the water. She was about to step out of the shower when she froze. Lindsay had come back into the bathroom. In her right hand she held a pair of scissors and in the other hand some new underwear that Jane had bought her for Christmas. Then she lashed out with the scissors, cutting the underwear into pieces. Jane was too terrified to move.

Lindsay then stormed back to her bedroom and slammed the door. Jane could hear her daughter as she swept through the room grabbing whatever she could and throwing it against the walls and the floor. The sound of breaking glass filled the house. Every present that Jane had given Lindsay—souvenir plates and cups, picture frames, even a tiny porcelain cheerleader—was being destroyed. Then Lindsay's door flew open again and she emerged wild-eyed and screaming as the rampage continued.

Beth Davies and Elizabeth Vines were in Pennington Gap attending a meeting when Jane Myers's sister came running into the room. She said that Jane had called to tell her that Lindsay had freaked out and that she needed Davies's help.

"My sister is going to die," she told the nun. "Her daughter is killing her."

Davies and Vines got into the woman's car and went speeding up to the Myerses' house. Once inside, it looked to Beth like a cyclone had hit. At first she couldn't find Jane. Then she finally saw her cowering in a corner. Lindsay then appeared. She looked high. As soon as Lindsay spotted Beth, she began to scream at her.

"Get out of my house!" she yelled. "Get out of my fucking house!"

A few minutes later Lindsay collapsed into a heap and started sobbing. Jane and Beth comforted her. When they got her settled down, Jane gave Lindsay a choice: she could go away to an inpatient treatment facility or she could stay at home and enter a methadone treatment program. Either way, Lindsay was told, her Oxy days were over.

CHAPTER SIX

HOT SPOTS

ART VAN ZEE WAS MAKING his rounds at Lee County Hospital one day in January 2001 when he ran into Vince Stravino in a corridor and stopped him. "You were right," he told Stravino about the need for a recall.

Van Zee was sickened by the devastation he had seen over the past year. His change of heart came after months of doubt. David Fiellin and Richard Schottenfeld, the Yale drug abuse treatment experts, had played a big role in his decision by pointing out that other drugs besides OxyContin could be used to treat patients with severe pain. Ultimately, however, it was the actions of Purdue executives—or their lack of action, in Van Zee's eyes—that sealed his decision. He believed that the drugmaker wasn't taking responsibility for the troubles its painkiller was causing and was determined to continue marketing it for general pain. Company executives like David Haddox had certainly dealt with him politely. But they'd shown no interest in limiting the drug's availability and had ignored his plea to send out an alert to doctors nationwide about the painkiller's increasing abuse.

As Van Zee drafted a petition demanding that the FDA recall OxyContin, flyers went out from the Lee Coalition for Health announcing a town meeting at Lee High in early March to discuss the area's OxyContin epidemic and the launch of a recall drive.

Meanwhile, at the beginning of March, just about a week before the Lee High gathering was scheduled, Purdue executives traveled to Richmond, Virginia, at the firm request of state Attorney General Mark Earley. In a letter to Purdue president Richard S. Sackler, Earley wrote that he wanted to discuss his "grave" concerns that the "widespread illegal sale of Oxy-Contin has created an epidemic of addiction and a surge in criminal behavior in Southwest Virginia."

Several company executives, though not Sackler himself, arrived in the state capital armed with a plan for combating the drug's abuse in Virginia. It contained elements of the drug abuse prevention program that Purdue had earlier announced in Maine, such as the distribution of tamper-resistant prescription pads. But the drugmaker also broadened the package to include an educational program aimed at alerting teenagers to the dangers of prescription drugs, and a $100,000 grant for a study to determine the best way to create a prescription monitoring system in Virginia.

One of the state officials who attended the meeting in Richmond was Gary Parsons, the Lee County sheriff. As he made the nearly seven-hour drive home, Parsons called Art Van Zee from his car to tell him about a conversation he'd had at the meeting's end with Purdue's top attorney, Howard Udell. The lawyer had mentioned to him that the pharmaceutical company was interested in making a donation to Lee County to help support drug abuse counseling programs.

A few days later, Parsons and Tammy McElyea, the state attorney for Lee County, dropped by the St. Charles clinic to talk about Purdue's plan with Van Zee, who took a break from seeing patients to meet with them. It was then that Parsons told Van Zee that it was his understanding that Purdue's offer to help the county had a string attached. Company officials did not want Van Zee to have anything to do with their money, Parsons said, because of his aggressive stance against their drug.

As Parsons later explained, "He was out advocating that the drug be taken off of the market and they were afraid that some of the money would be used to put out literature against their drug."

Van Zee told Parsons he didn't mind. "If it can help the county and I need to get left out, that's fine," he said, before going back to work.

A week or so later, Van Zee and Beth Davies stood on the same Lee High auditorium stage that Lindsay Myers had dragged herself across during the pep rally that had inaugurated

Senior Night. This time, though, the auditorium wasn't packed with cheering students but with about eight hundred adults distraught about a child, sibling, cousin, or friend whose life was ensnared in OxyContin abuse. Outside the school, a man clad in farmer's overalls had circulated through the crowd holding up a hastily scrawled cardboard sign that read: "Tell on Drug Pushers."

As they filed into the auditorium, hundreds of people signed Van Zee's recall petition. Jane Myers took a seat in the audience. So did Lindsay and Ray.

It was Lindsay's first trip back to Lee High in two months. Jane had pulled her out of school right after the horrific shower incident in January and, ever since, she and Ray had been making a daily four-hour round-trip to Knoxville, Tennessee, the site of the nearest methadone clinic. They started the drive at 1 A.M. so they could reach the clinic around 3:30 A.M. and nab a place near the front of the line. The clinic would open two hours later. The facility was located in a rough part of town; while they waited, dozing in Lindsay's car, dealers stood on nearby street corners selling crack cocaine.

Once inside, Lindsay waited for her number to be called. She was 3066. A receptionist then handed her a paper cup that she took with her into a bathroom. If her urine test showed she was free of drugs, she next went to a dosing room where a prescribed amount of methadone was poured into a plastic cup and mixed with water. To help improve the drug's flavor, Lindsay added some orange Gatorade, but it still tasted chalky and awful.

Lindsay decided to attend the town meeting at Lee High because she was trying hard to stick with her methadone program. Her situation at home had improved, and a teacher from the high school, hired by Jane, came every afternoon to the Myerses' house to teach Lindsay so she'd have a chance of graduating that spring with the rest of her class. Still, Lindsay couldn't help feeling that in taking methadone she was simply trading one drug for another.

Shortly after Lindsay took her seat in the back of the auditorium and the audience settled down, Sister Beth started the meeting.

"We are aware that many of you here tonight are carrying the heavy burden and indescribable pain of a loved one suffering from this chronic disease because addiction knows no boundaries," she said from the podium. "Others of you are desperately struggling to recover from the pain of addiction while trying to rebuild your lives. Unlike other diseases, persons who suffer from addiction often become alienated from their families, friends, and communities. As a community, we want to say to those who are suffering, all of you, we love you with the love that always welcomes you home."

Church leaders from nearby towns hard hit by the drug also offered faith as the way out of the despair caused by Oxy-Contin's abuse. "We can't help people after they are dead," the Reverend Ronnie Pennington of Hazard, Kentucky, declared. "We have to say we want our community back. A lot can be done as a group. God has the answers and the solutions."

Finally, Art Van Zee, who was not used to talking before

such a crowd, stood up to explain that he had set aside his initial reluctance to support a recall of the drug. For a time, he said, he had believed that the drug's benefits outweighed its risks, but now it was clear to him that its dangers were too great. "The pain and suffering brought to countless families and communities by the abuse of the drug surpass by an extraordinary degree its benefits," he said.

A report about the meeting took up most of the front page of the next edition of the *Powell Valley News,* the weekly newspaper published in Pennington Gap. The paper also published Purdue's response to the recall drive. In a letter to the editor, company officials pointed out that surveys at Lee High showed that students there were experimenting with many more drugs than just OxyContin, including marijuana, tranquilizers, and traditional painkillers like Percocet. The drugmaker was unequivocal in its opposition to a recall of OxyContin or any limitations on its use.

"Any effort to restrict access to OxyContin would be a disservice to the thousands of patients who rely on this medication to control their pain and regain function of their lives," the company's statement said.

It might seem unusual that a billion-dollar drug company like Purdue would feel it had anything to fear from a small-town doctor like Art Van Zee. But by early 2001, Purdue executives were beginning to feel a powerful backlash from the havoc caused by OxyContin.

Throughout much of the previous year, as Purdue executives like David Haddox traveled from one addiction-plagued community to another, they had told officials in various states that the painkiller's problems were limited to "hot spots," as they characterized areas hard hit by abuse. But in the late winter of 2001, Purdue was hit by a firestorm of bad publicity. The event that set it off was a massive drug raid in eastern Kentucky in February in which more than two hundred people were arrested on charges of illegally possessing or selling OxyContin. Dubbed "OxyFest" by law enforcement authorities, Kentucky officials called it the biggest drug sweep in their state's history.

Before the bust, coverage of the drug's problems had been largely limited to newspapers and television stations in badly afflicted areas. But the Kentucky drug bust turned OxyContin into big news, and reports about the raid were carried in national newspapers and on television networks.

Soon the national news media seized on OxyContin as the tale of a "wonder" drug gone awry, a high-powered and supposedly abuse-resistant painkiller that had become a street drug tearing communities apart. A few weeks after OxyFest, a lengthy, front-page article in the *New York Times* raised questions about Purdue's safety claims for OxyContin and reported that some doctors and pharmacists believed the drugmaker had contributed to the problem by marketing its painkiller too aggressively. In addition, coroners and other local authorities cited in the *Times* estimated that OxyContin had been a factor in at least 120 drug overdose deaths. One Drug Enforcement Administration official was quoted as saying that no other prescription drug introduced since the early 1980s had been abused by so many people so soon after it had gone on the market.

Other major articles appeared in weekly newsmagazines including *Time*, *Newsweek*, and even *People*. A public relations firm hired by Purdue to monitor and analyze news coverage of OxyContin reported to the company in March that "Oxy-Contin stories continue to permeate the media." Numerous examples were cited, including one report on the NBC television network that typified the tone of the media coverage:

On March 22, the NBC "Evening News" aired a segment focusing on the abuse of OxyContin among teenagers and young adults. While NBC's report provided fairly balanced coverage, it was led by a teaser on a number of local NBC affiliates, in some of the nation's biggest media markets, incorporating the story of a woman whose OxyContin-addicted husband tried to burn their house down. In her own words, "[T]hem things should be taken off the market. They are killing people." In the NBC "Evening News" national report, a physician said he won't prescribe OxyContin to his patients and suggests that the drug should be reformulated to make it less addictive. These statements are the kinds of statements that provide fire for legislators looking to regulate the prescribing patterns of physicians and, as a result of NBC's coverage, people all over the country heard them.

Only months before, most reporters had never heard of Oxy-Contin or Purdue. Little also was known about the Sacklers, the extraordinarily wealthy family who owned Purdue. And even those who recognized the Sackler name were less likely to connect it with pharmaceuticals than with the galleries the family had underwritten in art museums worldwide, including the Metropolitan Museum of Art in New York City and the Smithsonian in Washington, D.C. While photographs of family members appeared from time to time in society page coverage of museum benefits, they scrupulously avoided being interviewed about their business interests.

Upon first hearing of Purdue, some people mistakenly think the company has some connection to Purdue University; in fact, the Sacklers had simply taken over the name Purdue Frederick from a tiny drugmaker in New York City that they had purchased in 1952. Unlike most major pharmaceutical companies in the United States such as Merck and Johnson & Johnson, whose stock is publicly traded, the drugmaker was privately held by the family. That meant that its financial records and business dealings weren't open to inspection by outsiders such as Wall Street analysts or investors. The drugmaker also wasn't required to file reports with the federal Securities and Exchange Commission, which regulates the financial disclosures of publicly traded concerns. As a result, reporters didn't cover the company; drug industry analysts didn't opine about its operations; and outside directors, who serve on the boards of publicly traded companies, didn't influence its decisions. Purdue was the Sackler family's private domain.

Used to operating in anonymity, company executives and Sackler family members found the steady barrage of news coverage a shock. But now, even as the drugmaker faced its greatest crisis, the company's two surviving founders, brothers Dr. Raymond Sackler and Dr. Mortimer Sackler—both well into their eighties at the time—remained behind the scenes. Raymond's son Richard, who was Purdue's president, also made no public comments about the painkiller's abuse. When they needed to say something to the world, be it to government officials or the news media, the Sacklers allowed executives like Haddox or Michael Friedman, the drugmaker's chief operating officer, to serve as the public face of their company.

In mid-March of 2001 the drugmaker had other problems on its hands besides the news media. FDA officials, alarmed by what they were reading or seeing in television reports, contacted Purdue headquarters and in a teleconference with top company executives expressed their concerns. "It was made very clear to them that we were greatly concerned about what we were hearing and we wanted to know how we could work together and intercede before the problem got worse," an FDA official later recalled.

Suddenly, the fate of OxyContin and the fortunes of Purdue itself hung in the balance as the company and FDA officials entered into what would become months of delicate discussions about the drug's future. It was a marked departure from only a year before. In early 2000, Richard Sackler had told a gathering of sales reps that he anticipated that OxyContin's remarkable sales growth would continue to fuel the drugmaker for years to come. "OxyContin tablets have by no means run their course," he told them. "There is no sign of it slowing down."

Now, instead, Purdue executives found the company's reputation under attack and their own decisions questioned by government regulators and the news media. "We were getting creamed, we were getting killed," the head of Purdue's public relations staff, Robin Hogen, later told a gathering of professionals in his field. "It was like being a prizefighter and you were getting punched in the stomach, and then in the cheek, and then in the stomach again, and you're sort of reeling. We were on the ropes with this kind of coverage on a product that creates about 80 percent of our revenue."

As the media whirlwind gathered in early 2001, the drugmaker hired a small battalion of corporate crisis management experts and media consultants to supplement its own small internal public relations staff. Based in Washington, D.C., the McGinn Group previously had represented embattled breast implant manufacturers and the lead paint industry. Nichols/Dezenhall, another Washington firm hired by Purdue, called itself "the leader in crisis management and high-stakes communication." The mission of the two firms was to calm the roiling waters surrounding OxyContin and to launch a counterattack against what Purdue officials felt were unfair depictions of the company's practices in publications including the *New York Times*.

A multipronged counteroffensive emerged that apparently was intended to reinforce the legitimate use of OxyContin while deflecting the media's focus away from the painkiller and onto the issue of prescription drug abuse in general. As Purdue officials would soon put it, their product had simply become the latest "drug du jour" in a long line of abused medications. In support of their case, company officials produced graphic pie charts intended to show that the number of overdose reports involving hydrocodone-containing painkillers like Vicodin was far higher than that involving oxycodone-containing drugs like OxyContin.

But at the center of Purdue's defense of OxyContin were pain patients and the ways in which the drug improved their lives. Carefully coached by hired consultants, company executives lectured reporters and government regulators that it was unthinkable that the irresponsible acts of drug abusers should jeopardize the access of legitimate patients to the medication they needed. They argued that the news media's focus on the drug's dark side had exacerbated the problems that pain patients faced. In early 2001 a small Virginia public relations firm, one of many local concerns hired by Purdue to combat its problems in states with particularly bad abuse problems, described its mission as helping Purdue get "out the message that patients with pain are the 'silent victims' of all the press coverage of OxyContin abuse."

There was little question that the growing coverage of the painkiller's abuse was having some ripple effects on patient treatment, though how much was impossible to quantify. Some doctors reduced their prescriptions of OxyContin or stopped dispensing it altogether. And some patients, concerned by reports that highlighted the drug's addictive potential, asked doctors to take them off the painkiller even though they had been doing well on it.

Soon some articles appeared warning, as others had done at the start of the pain management movement, that a new "war on drugs" was threatening the well-being of pain patients. In a column that appeared in *Electronic Media*, a trade publication, Tom Shales, a television critic, suggested in early 2001 that the intense media coverage of OxyContin was causing the curious to experiment with the drug. Newscasts "tell you how to get high. Then the correspondents do follow-up reports expressing shock and dismay that the abuse is becoming more popular," wrote Shales, who also worked as a television critic for the *Washington Post*. "Yeah, more kids are using the drug to get high because they heard about it and even saw how to use it on the evening news."

Meanwhile, David Haddox and other top executives at Purdue started meeting with newspaper editorial boards to present their case. Purdue, they said, had moved as quickly as possible when it first learned of the drug's abuse to curtail it by undertaking programs like the plan it had unveiled in Virginia. In fact, Purdue officials said, the abuse prevention efforts launched by the company were without precedent in the pharmaceutical industry. They were setting what they called "a new standard in corporate responsibility."

In March 2001, about a week after the town meeting at Lee High, Art Van Zee received a call from Purdue. A staffer asked whether Van Zee would meet with a contingent of top company executives if they flew to Lee County to see him. Van Zee said he'd be happy to do so. When he told Sue Ella about the phone call that evening, however, an alarm inside her went off. Purdue hadn't told Art why they wanted to see him, and she worried that company officials planned to use the meeting to discuss the recall petition. She feared they might even threaten to sue Art if he didn't withdraw it.

Years before, Sue Ella, while representing a local environmental group, had been sued for $10 million by a waste disposal company that wanted to dump New York City garbage in Appalachia. The company's lawsuit, as well as its garbage dumping plan, had failed. But she remembered how the company had used the lawsuit as a weapon against a much weaker opponent, and the lawyer in Sue Ella feared Purdue might try a similar preemptive strike against her husband. She didn't want Art to go by himself to meet with the Purdue team, and other members of the Lee Coalition for Health agreed.

So on a late March afternoon, three cars full of coalition members left Pennington Gap for the nearby town of Duffield, where the drug company's executives were expecting to meet alone with Van Zee at a Ramada Inn. Along with Van Zee and Sue Ella Kobak, those making the short drive included Beth Davies, Elizabeth Vines, Larry Lavender, Vince Stravino, and Greg Stewart.

When the group entered the motel's lobby, it was empty. Then a woman approached Beth Davies.

"Hello, Sister Davies," she said.

Beth didn't recognize her. "How do you know me?" she asked.

The woman explained that she worked for Purdue and had attended the Lee High meeting. She then told the group that the company's corporate jet had been delayed taking off from Connecticut, but that she expected her colleagues momentarily.

About an hour later the Purdue team arrived, led by David Haddox. He shook hands with Van Zee and Lavender and then introduced his colleagues: Howard Udell, the lawyer, and Michael Friedman, Purdue's chief operating officer. During the past year it had been Haddox, Udell, and Friedman who had played the leading public roles for Purdue in its dealing with state and local officials.

Udell was a short, portly man with a sagging double chin who in 2001 was sixty, though he looked older. He had spent much of his legal career working for the Sackler family, first at a New York City law firm that handled much of its legal work and later at Purdue. Udell could be extremely gracious and projected a grandfatherly image. But he was also a very shrewd and aggressive lawyer playing a critical role in steering Purdue through the storm surrounding OxyContin.

Friedman, who was tall with curly red hair and a mustache, had as his principal responsibilities sales and marketing. Before working in the pharmaceutical industry he had spent many years as a top marketing executive for Hilti International, a manufacturer of industrial bolts and construction fasteners; he then became chief executive of Castolin Eutectic, a company in the welding and metal treatment business. The story that circu-

lated around Purdue headquarters was that Friedman and
Richard Sackler, the son of a Purdue founder, in the mid-1980s
were seated next to each other on an airplane flight. The two
men struck up a conversation and Sackler was so impressed by
Friedman that he offered him a job. Friedman first was responsible for seeking licensing deals for the drugmaker, and he eventually started working his way up through the company's sales
and marketing operation. In the late 1990s, he was given the
title of chief operating officer, and Friedman proclaimed in
1999 that it was his "vision" that Purdue's growth over the
next decade would be so spectacular that it would join the
ranks of the ten largest pharmaceutical companies in the United
States.

At the time of the meeting at the Ramada Inn in Duffield,
Friedman and Udell had every reason to feel like they were
under siege. Only two weeks had passed, for instance, since
FDA officials had contacted the drugmaker about the Oxy-
Contin abuse problems. The company had also recently met
with DEA officials. Still, as they shook hands with the contingent from Lee County, both Udell and Friedman appeared relaxed.

"We understand you folks are having a horrible problem,"
those at the meeting recalled Friedman as saying. "We are here
to see what we can do to help."

He then recounted the measures that Purdue already had
taken to cut down on OxyContin's misuse. He added that the
company had begun to work directly with affected local communities, even funding drug counseling services in some areas.

The drugmaker was considering underwriting a similar program in Lee County, Friedman explained, carefully emphasizing that the decision to offer such aid would go forward even if the Lee Coalition continued to pursue its recall petition. He didn't mention anything about excluding Art Van Zee.

Friedman struck those present as courteous and concerned. But Van Zee and the others were unmoved; if Purdue wanted to help, they said, the company should stop promoting Oxy-Contin for noncancer pain until it was reformulated. Purdue had recently announced that it had started investigating ways to make the painkiller more resistant to abuse, but David Haddox retorted that to withdraw it now from the market would only harm patients who needed it.

As the two sides advanced toward a predictable stalemate, Vince Stravino began to boil. He believed that places like Lee County were only OxyContin's first stops on its march of destruction. Stravino explained to the Purdue executives that neither he nor Van Zee had a stake in the OxyContin fight. Nobody in Lee County had anything to gain or lose from Oxy-Contin either financially or professionally. They simply were trying to open the company's eyes. Before long, it wouldn't just be the overdosed teenage sons and daughters of poor parents in Appalachia who'd be turning up dead in emergency rooms, Stravino warned. Soon kids from affluent, suburban homes would start dying. And their parents wouldn't hesitate to sue Purdue, embroiling it in ugly and expensive litigation for years to come.

"The genie is out of the bottle," he angrily told the company's executives. "This is only the beginning. This is going to follow you everywhere."

Van Zee had brought another man to the meeting as well, a local bank official who up until that moment had not spoken. After the physician had introduced him, the man took out photographs of his family and showed them to Purdue's executives. He talked proudly about his daughter, a successful teacher. Then he told Haddox, Udell, and Friedman a personal tale of the misery caused by OxyContin's misuse.

All his family happiness, he said, had gotten squeezed out of his life after his youngest son became hooked on Oxys. It was an all-too-typical story: First, things that could be easily sold, like tools and guns, had disappeared from the family's home. Then huge credit card bills run up by his son arrived. His son kept denying there was a problem, and the worried father, much like Jane Myers with Lindsay, didn't know what to do. The boy kept getting worse until finally, when it seemed like his life was in the balance, he agreed to seek help. Two years later, his son was barely hanging on. His OxyContin habit and ongoing treatment had already cost the family about eighty thousand dollars, all but depleting their retirement savings. When he'd finished his story, he told Friedman, Udell, and Haddox that he agreed with Dr. Van Zee; he thought Purdue should take the drug off the market until it could be made safer.

"We are an average American family," the man said. "Surely you have got enough patriotism to worry about this country?"

The Purdue group remained silent during the man's story.

Finally, Michael Friedman spoke. "I'm sorry your family is having such a problem," he said.

The meeting was about to break up when Howard Udell picked his briefcase off the floor and opened it. He removed several large pieces of paper and passed them around.

"I want to show you this because it's going to run in the local newspaper," he explained.

The pages were photocopies of a full-page newspaper advertisement. The ad's headline read: "An Open Letter to the Citizens of Lee County from Purdue Pharma." At its end, the "letter" bore David Haddox's name, as though it were a personal note from him.

"I am a native of Appalachia and a physician who has spent much of my life studying and treating both pain and drug abuse," the ad read. "But today I am writing to you on behalf of Purdue Pharma L.P., the company that manufactures Oxy-Contin Tablets."

Haddox's letter went on to say that Purdue was greatly concerned about "the devastation that prescription drug abuse is having on Lee County" and was committed to addressing it. However, the company wanted to "clarify some information that was discussed at the recent meetings at Lee County High School so that we can work together from a platform of truth."

The ad stated in boldfaced type that it was absolutely untrue that Purdue had targeted its marketing of OxyContin to areas like Appalachia with high disability or Medicaid rates. "It is equally false to say that Purdue knew about the abuse potential of OxyContin from the beginning and did nothing about it," the advertisement stated. It also disputed suggestions that a reformulation of OxyContin by Purdue would be quick or easy.

"We understand that Lee County residents are about to expend great effort and energy to promote a petition demanding the recall of OxyContin," the ad continued. "We are fortunate to live in a country where we can all express our views openly. However, we are concerned that the problem of abuse will not be solved by removal of a single drug, particularly one that millions of patients depend upon. . . . Instead of this futile petition drive, the energies of the people of Lee County could be spent on positive ways of dealing with the terrible problem of drug abuse and addiction" through efforts that included school education programs and prescription monitoring plans.

To both Vince Stravino and Beth Davies, the whole meeting now suddenly seemed like a setup orchestrated by Purdue executives to shove the ad down their throats. But it was Sue Ella who exploded, turning her anger on Haddox.

"This is the most insulting thing that I have ever seen," she told him. "You have done more to hurt Appalachia than the coal industry has ever thought about doing."

Haddox sat bolt upright. "I resent that," he said.

"I don't give a damn if you do," she replied. "The truth will stand. I am not going to stay here."

She stormed out into the lobby. Greg Stewart, the pharmacist, soon joined her.

"I'm going to pay the bill," she told him.

"I've already paid it," he said.

"Did you pay for theirs too?" Sue Ella asked.

"Hell, no," Stewart replied.

The following morning, three Purdue executives gathered at Kathy's Country Kitchen, a small café in Jonesville, the Lee County seat, for a meeting with several local officials including Sheriff Parsons and Tammy McElyea, the public prosecutor. Beth Davies was there too, and when she looked across the table at David Haddox he seemed to be still sulking as a result of the previous evening's meeting. For their part, Friedman and Udell listened as Sheriff Parsons and others described how the area's limited drug treatment and law enforcement resources had been overwhelmed by OxyContin's abuse.

"Maybe we could help," Friedman offered.

"How much could you afford?" an official asked.

Friedman and Udell responded that the drugmaker would be happy to contribute a hundred thousand dollars. Many at the table enthusiastically greeted the offer. Sister Beth, however, shot Udell a look.

After they left, the drug company officials apparently had second thoughts about the wisdom of David Haddox's "open letter" to the people of Lee County, because it never appeared in the newspaper. Meanwhile, the Lee Coalition for Health had to decide what to do about the offer from Purdue. At a series of meetings, several members, including Sheriff Parsons and Greg Stewart, said they thought the group should accept the money.

Stewart said that since Purdue had made a small fortune from the area's misery it ought to give some of it back to repair the damage. Van Zee was of a similar mind, and he drafted a letter from the coalition accepting Purdue's funds.

Sister Beth made sure it was never sent. She told Van Zee and the others that she'd quit the coalition if it took the company's money. She said she was sick of seeing corporate executives flying into Appalachia with their olive branch checkbooks as a way of putting out firestorms and buying peace. Businesses had been doing it for years: mining companies, logging companies, garbage haulers. This time it was a drug company. But regardless of what the companies were selling or doing, their goals were always the same, she said. Their executives all asked "What can we do for you?" but what they really wanted was for their problems to go away.

Well, this time that wasn't going to happen, she insisted. Too many lives already had been destroyed. Yes, the money might do some good, but Purdue would get something far more valuable in return, Beth argued: their name for its public relations machine.

"This is blood money and we aren't going to take it," she said. "They're trying to buy us off."

No one argued with Sister Beth.

CHAPTER SEVEN

KIDDIE DOPE

DAVID HADDOX, MICHAEL Friedman, and Howard Udell were escorted to a conference room on the sixth floor of one of the twin black-glass office buildings that house the federal Drug Enforcement Administration in Arlington, Virginia. There, they were greeted by Laura Nagel, a tall and thin woman with a narrow face framed by untamed dirty-blond hair, who headed a section of the agency known as the Office of Diversion Control. As its name implies, one of the unit's jobs was to prevent prescription narcotics and other controlled substances from ending up on the street.

Nagel had just come to the diversion section when the Oxy-Contin crisis exploded. Until a few months before the Purdue contingent's visit to the DEA in early 2001, she had worked as an agent and then a supervisor in the agency's bigger and better-known criminal division. That unit has long been the federal government's principal weapon in its war against traffickers in illicit drugs. Along with a stint in San Francisco, Nagel had worked as a criminal agent in New York and Phoenix before she started her rise through the agency's hierarchy. Now, with her recent promotion at the end of 2000 to the head of the diversion division, Nagel, at the age of forty-three, had become one of highest-ranking women at DEA.

She had gotten her first inklings about the abuse of Oxy-Contin in late 2000 from fellow law enforcement officials in West Virginia. But it was only after the "OxyFest" bust that winter and the subsequent torrent of news stories that the size of the problem became clear to her. Nagel wasn't the type of person who'd shy away from either making a decision or getting involved in a fight. She quickly called together some long-time diversion unit staffers to help her assess the situation. By early March, they had reached a consensus. They believed that Purdue's claim that OxyContin was less prone to abuse was wrong. And they also decided that the drugmaker hadn't done enough to alert doctors and other health professionals about the drug's problems. As a result, doctors had prescribed the narcotic too freely and too much of it was winding up on the street. The situation had become so grave that a DEA official told the *New York Times* in early March, "It may take years to repair the damage that this drug has done."

A few days after that article appeared, Michael Friedman

wrote to Nagel to set up a meeting. "We are writing as a consequence of the recent and widespread news reports concerning the illegal diversion and abuse in various areas of the country of one of this Company's analgesic products, OxyContin," Friedman wrote.

> We take this problem very seriously, as it is reminiscent of other events that have taken place over the years as new opioids have become available. The criminal element seems always able to devise means to evade the legal protective mechanisms that have been put in place and which are observed fully and conscientiously by the great bulk of licensed manufacturers, distributors and prescribers.
>
> Purdue Pharma has been working actively during the past year with federal, state and local officials to assist in their efforts for dealing with this drug diversion and abuse problem. We initiated a series of major programs to assure the OxyContin tablets are used in an appropriate and lawful manner. Purdue believes that these initiatives are important because OxyContin Tablets and other legal opioid-containing drugs are of critical importance for providing relief to numerous patients in moderate to severe pain.

It was David Haddox who began the company's presentation to Nagel and other DEA officials on that day in late March. He turned on a laptop computer and launched a PowerPoint program that projected slides of graphics onto the wall. Haddox's talk, like many similar ones he had given before, was centered on the inadequate treatment of pain and the recent drive by the medical community to use narcotics to treat it more aggressively. Purdue executives also explained what the company had done to try to curtail OxyContin's misuse.

Haddox's presentation struck Nagel as a slickly produced dog and pony show. She let him continue for a few minutes, then asked him to shut off the computer so they could talk about the drug's abuse.

"This has gotten out of control," she said. "We need to do something."

She started throwing out some ideas she had gotten from members of her staff. Nagel suggested, for instance, that given the growing number of drugstore robberies, it might be useful to restrict dispensing the product at a limited number of drugstores in each town or city. She also asked Purdue to consider limiting the drug's prescribing privileges to only those doctors who were trained or certified in pain treatment. She told Haddox, Friedman, and Udell that the agency believed that the painkiller's wide availability had made it an easy target for drug abusers and recreational users.

The Purdue executives listened politely. They didn't voice any opinions about Nagel's suggestions. "We'll take that under advisement," Howard Udell told her, leaving it at that.

Nagel also mentioned that she was greatly disturbed by newspaper accounts concerning overdose deaths, as well as reports that Purdue sales reps had pushed OxyContin too hard.

Those articles had quoted some doctors as saying that Purdue sales reps had tried to convince them to use OxyContin for insignificant injuries, and druggists had also been quoted as saying that they had been told by reps that they might get sued by patients if they didn't fill OxyContin prescriptions. Friedman and Udell said the company was looking into the overdose reports but they refuted any marketing excesses, emphasizing that they believed Purdue's sales policies to be extremely "conservative" by pharmaceutical industry standards. Nonetheless, they invited Nagel to alert them to any specific cases where a sales rep may have overstepped proper bounds so they could investigate.

After the Purdue team left the building, Nagel told one colleague that the meeting had been an incredible waste of time. The company hadn't agreed to do anything.

About ten days later she received a five-page letter from Michael Friedman. Its central theme was that the news media and other critics of OxyContin had exaggerated the number of overdose deaths in which the drug might have played a role and inaccurately portrayed how Purdue had marketed the drug. "Purdue is working to gather information to help us understand the media reports of abuse, diversion and death attributed to OxyContin Tablets," Friedman wrote on April 2.

> As we discussed at the meeting, we do not want to minimize the significance of even one death; however, a clear understanding of the scope of the problem will help us all to better define how to deal with the problem. Prior to

our meeting, we had received media reports of 59 deaths in Kentucky, 35 deaths in Maine, 20 deaths in Pennsylvania, and 28 deaths in Virginia. As you know, we are required to research all reported incidents of death and report our findings to FDA. This is what we know thus far:

• We have obtained a letter from the State Medical Examiner's Office in Kentucky. This letter (March 1, 2001) states that " . . . I am unaware of any reliable data in Kentucky that proves that OxyContin is causing a lot of deaths. In the State M.E. Office, we are seeing an increase in the number of deaths from ingesting several different prescription drugs and mixing them with alcohol. OxyContin is sometimes one of these drugs."

• We have obtained data from the Office of the Chief Medical Examiner in Maine. This data reports that during 1999 and part of 2000, there were 12 overdose deaths in which oxycodone was identified. Oxycodone was the sole chemical identified in only two cases, one of which was a suicide.

• As of this writing, we have only been able to obtain data from one county in Pennsylvania, Blair. . . . In this county, which encompasses Altoona, during the period from January 13, 1996 to December 1, 2000, there were 58 reported "Drug Deaths." Of these deaths, seven involved oxycodone as one of the agents causing death due to multiple drug toxicity. In no case was oxycodone listed as a single cause of death. We have no information at this point as to whether any of these deaths involved OxyContin.

• We are attempting to obtain data on the reported deaths in western Virginia involving oxycodone. We were told by one of the medical examiners in The Chief Medical Examiners Office of Virginia that there had been 31, not 28 deaths in western Virginia since 1997 involving oxycodone. Unfortunately, the authorities have not complied with our requests for information on the reported deaths. We have asked Attorney General Earley to help us obtain this information. At our meeting, you indicated that DEA might be able to obtain this information. We request that if you are able to do so, you consider sharing that information with us.

• As you can see, the facts that we have been able to obtain thus far are quite different than the media reports. We are not suggesting that there is no abuse and diversion. In fact, we know that such diversion and abuse exists. We just need to know how much, where and the source of diverted materials, so that we can all properly address the problem. As we discussed, we will send you summaries of our reports to the FDA on all of these cases. We would also appreciate any information that you can provide to us.

In his letter, Friedman rejected any suggestions that Purdue had inappropriately marketed OxyContin. The Purdue executive added that he believed much of the criticism had come from doctors who didn't believe that the use of opioids for moderate or severe pain was acceptable medical practice. He also said that the company believed that Nagel's suggestion of limiting the number of pharmacies that could dispense OxyContin was impractical and would create hardships for pain patients. Friedman, however, acknowledged concerns that drug runners might be buying OxyContin at pharmacies in Mexico or Canada and smuggling it into the United States. As a result, he wrote, Purdue had decided to put special markings on tablets shipped to Mexico so that law enforcement authorities would know that the pills came from Mexico if they were seized during drug busts in this country. The company had also modified its sales bonus plan to encourage reps to "sell to a broad base of doctors rather than focus on any single physician," his letter stated.

"I believe that we made great progress at our meeting in improving our understanding of this situation," Friedman wrote, in conclusion. "Purdue would like to continue to work with the DEA to stop the abuse and diversion of OxyContin and help address the broader problem of prescription drug abuse."

Friedman's letter was the start of a trail of bad blood between Laura Nagel and Purdue. His response, several DEA officials would later say, infuriated her because she viewed it as the drug company's declaration that it was prepared to battle her every step of the way.

"It's a screw-you letter," she told one colleague.

In many ways, OxyContin turned the DEA's traditional view of the drug world on its head. Cases involving legal pharmaceutical substances such as OxyContin had always been seen as less important than those involving illegal drugs—that's why hard-charging criminal agents referred derisively to prescription drugs as "kiddie dope." Also, diversion investigators played second fiddle to criminal agents on the agency's career ladder. Along with earning lower retirement benefits, they weren't permitted to carry guns or conduct undercover operations. If they wanted to seize medical records from a doctor suspected of running a pill mill, they had to ask a DEA criminal agent to serve the search warrant.

But with OxyContin it was suddenly clear that a legal drug could be as devastating in terms of deaths and crime as any illicit substance. For instance, a little more than a month after Purdue executives met with Laura Nagel, state officials in Florida announced that during the second half of 2000 threre were more overdose deaths in the state from prescription narcotics like OxyContin and Vicodin than from heroin and cocaine.

Still, as Laura Nagel and other agency officials tried to address the issue of OxyContin abuse, they realized that the DEA was ill equipped to deal with a problem of its magnitude.

During the previous decade, the diversion division had been decimated as a result of events both inside and outside the agency. Both manpower and morale had hit a low point. In the 1990s drug agents had been a favorite whipping boy of pain management advocates, who depicted them in much the same way that gun lovers portrayed firearms agents—as jackbooted thugs who ripped prescription pads out of the hands of well-meaning doctors.

In reality, the diversion office was a beaten and toothless watchdog. Its investigators were so dizzied by the medical profession's sudden and rapid acceptance of narcotics that their jobs seemed superfluous at times. By the end of the 1990s the DEA's diversion office had all but given up investigating doctors for illegally prescribing narcotics. The DEA routinely approved the big production hikes sought by narcotics makers and frequently appeared at events put on by pharmaceutical companies like Purdue to help doctors understand how to stay on the right side of the law when they prescribed narcotics. For instance, an agency official spoke at meetings put on by the Appalachian Pain Foundation. Hit by a tidal wave of change, the diversion unit had learned to swim with the tide.

The section also had been undermined from within the DEA. Its problems began in 1994 with the appointment of Thomas Constantine as the agency's new administrator. During his five-year tenure, Constantine, a former New York State Police Department superintendent, was disliked within the agency, according to a 1995 report in *U.S. News & World Report*. His harsh style caused many top criminal agents to leave. But while the ranks of the criminal-side staff doubled during his tenure, Constantine had little use for the agency's prescription drug operation, and employees of the unit said he considered them to be little more than meddlesome regulators.

Constantine once told a group of drug company executives

that he understood their impatience with regulators because he had similar frustrations while heading the New York State police, according to a former DEA official who attended the meeting.

"Those regulators from OSHA used to come into my barracks and check to see if the shoe polish was edible," Constantine said, referring to the federal Occupational Safety and Health Administration.

When one diversion division official protested the unit's treatment, Constantine spelled out his bottom line.

"Has a diversion investigator ever been killed in the line of duty?" he wanted to know. The conversation ended when he was told that none had.

By the time Constantine left DEA in 1999, the battering had taken its toll. The diversion division was rudderless and dispirited and many of its staffers alienated.

Laura Nagel had never met Art Van Zee. Their personalities couldn't have been more different. While Van Zee was soft-spoken and knew little about the workings of Washington, Nagel, who had grown up in the suburbs of New York City, was blunt and politically adept. Still, as the spring of 2001 progressed, Nagel shared Van Zee's weariness with the constant public avowals coming from Purdue executives that their actions on the OxyContin front had been guided by the public's interests rather than the company's quest for profits.

She also saw Purdue's characterization of OxyContin as just

another "drug du jour" as self-serving. She believed quite the opposite, that the painkiller was unique and the forerunner of a new generation of high-powered painkillers already in the pharmaceutical industry's pipeline that could produce similar chaos if let loose without added safeguards. In 1999, Purdue itself had announced plans to market a timed-release version of Dilaudid, the powerful synthetic narcotic that had earned the nickname "drugstore heroin" when it first appeared in the 1920s. The company was already selling the painkiller in Canada, but the FDA found problems with Purdue's application and delayed approving its sales in the United States.

But Nagel, unlike Art Van Zee, remained opposed to recalling OxyContin. Van Zee believed that there were less-abuse-prone alternatives available. It was Nagel's feeling, however, that there weren't sufficient legal grounds for a recall and that the threat posed by the painkiller could be sharply reduced if Purdue stopped promoting it for moderate pain, a step that would make it far less available. It was clear to her, however, that Purdue took a very different view of things. And Nagel decided that she wasn't about to wait for Purdue executives to change their minds. So she began to put pressure on Purdue in another forum—the court of public opinion.

In early May 2001 the DEA announced the start of a sweeping program to reduce the abuse of OxyContin. Agency officials described the initiative as the first time that the DEA had targeted a specific brand-name prescription drug, rather than a class of medications, for special attention.

Laura Nagel knew that she could be hotheaded—even volatile at times—so she assigned one of her top aides, Terrance Woodworth, a longtime diversion division official, to act as her public voice on the issue of OxyContin. Soon, Woodworth, who was known as Terry, started giving interviews challenging Purdue to voluntarily restrict its marketing effort and urging the company to drop its contention that OxyContin was less likely to be abused than similar narcotics.

For instance, Woodworth told the *New York Times* in May 2001 that agency officials believed Purdue's promotion of Oxy-Contin was causing physicians to use it without first trying milder drugs.

"DEA is extremely concerned that many doctors are prescribing this strong narcotic as an initial treatment for many types of pain," he said.

Before long, Terry Woodworth was squaring off against David Haddox on television news and talk show segments devoted to the drug's problems.

"The abuse and diversion [of OxyContin] has just skyrocketed in various communities, from Maine to Florida, all along the East Coast," Woodworth said on the *Early Show*, a CBS morning talk program. "And it's moving into the central United States. We're getting reports from Arizona and Nevada, Washington and Oregon, and even Alaska is reporting a growing abuse problem."

Haddox acknowledged that there had been some instances of abuse, but he insisted that the focus needed to remain on pain patients and their needs. "I think that one of the nice things about medicine in this country is that doctors have a lot of choices," he told the same interviewer. "And what you've heard thus far this morning on the segment is the problems with abuse of the drug. No one's talked about the patients. There are 50 million patients in this country who have chronic pain that's not being managed appropriately every single day. OxyContin is one of the choices that doctors have available to them to treat that."

The public and Purdue weren't the only intended audience for Nagel's campaign; she also wanted to goad FDA officials into taking decisive action. In the realm of prescription drugs, the jobs performed by the DEA and the FDA are supposed to complement each other, but the agencies' differing mandates said much about the dilemma OxyContin posed to regulators: how to keep the drug out of the wrong hands while keeping it available to pain patients. As long as FDA officials were convinced that OxyContin wasn't harming legitimate pain patients, they were under no immediate pressure to take action. Purdue and FDA officials had started negotiations in late March about what steps to take to halt the painkiller's misuse, but Nagel worried as those talks continued that drug regulators wouldn't go far enough.

In the late spring of 2001, as Laura Nagel continued to step up the pressure on Purdue, company public relations strategists began suggesting to reporters that the DEA was unfairly beating up on the drugmaker to enhance its own prestige. It was also around that same time that Nagel was alerted by colleagues at the Justice Department—the federal department that oversees the DEA—that Purdue executives had arranged a meeting with one of her superiors through a political lobbyist.

Nagel saw the move as an effort by Purdue to make an end run around her; so did Justice Department officials, who invited her to the meeting without notifying Purdue. When Michael Friedman and Howard Udell walked into a conference room at Justice Department headquarters in Washington, they appeared surprised to see Nagel, although Udell quickly recovered.

"We were going to stop in and see you while we were in town," he said with a smile.

The importance of the Justice Department meeting to Purdue was signaled by the presence of Richard Sackler. It was one of the first times that Sackler had ventured out from the company's Stamford headquarters to defend OxyContin before government officials.

Like his father and his uncle, Sackler, who was fifty-six in 2001, had trained as a physician before entering the family's drug business. He was known around Purdue headquarters as a pleasant man, though he appeared uncomfortable at times in groups of people. For example, while he annually addressed the company's sales force, he rarely stayed afterward to mingle. And those who did business with Purdue were left with the strong impression that Richard Sackler played a secondary role; Mortimer and Raymond Sackler, it seemed, still made the big decisions despite their advanced ages.

Now, at the Justice Department meeting, Richard Sackler was dressed casually in a tweed sports jacket and a shirt with a button-down collar. As he took his seat in the conference room,

Laura Nagel passed her business card across the table to him and he lined it up on the table's edge alongside the other cards he had received.

Purdue's executives assured the Justice Department officials that they had taken proper steps to promote OxyContin and now were doing everything possible to curb its abuse. Richard Sackler didn't speak much during the gathering, although he broke into the company's formal presentation at one point to remark that OxyContin was an extremely good drug.

Nagel didn't doubt that for a minute, although she remained convinced that Purdue should do more to help prevent its abuse. She decided to use the meeting as an opportunity to appeal directly to Richard Sackler because he was both a doctor and member of a family well known for its philanthropic contributions to the arts and to medical institutions. She also wanted him to understand that if he didn't do more, she would.

At one point, Nagel leaned across the table, bringing her face closer to his.

"People are dying, do you understand that?" she told him. "And I'm not going to back down."

Sackler looked shaken for a moment and then stared down at the business cards in front of him.

"I think I understand that," he replied.

It wasn't long before Purdue moved to counter the DEA's criticisms of the company and its drug. In June 2001, for instance, Howard Udell wrote to Nagel to alert her that the newspaper

USA Today was about to publish an editorial about Oxy-Contin. In his letter, Udell quoted directly from a message he had just received from James Heins, who worked in the drug-maker's public relations office.

"*USA Today* is planning an editorial on how DEA is handling the OxyContin abuse and diversion issue," Heins' message to Udell began. "It will probably appear on Wednesday of this week. Based on conversations that I and David Haddox had with the writer, it appears that the piece will be critical of the DEA's actions. Both David and I took pain to avoid taking an adversarial position to the DEA."

The tone of the *USA Today* editorial was captured by the headline: "DEA Overreaches in Effort to Stop Abuse of Painkiller." It stated that the agency's proposals to limit the pre-scribing of OxyContin to pain specialists would harm patients because there were only four thousand such specialists in the country. And it argued that the DEA's singular focus on Oxy-Contin's role was misguided because forty other prescription drugs also contained oxycodone as their active ingredient.

"More importantly, there's little evidence that restricting pa-tients' access to painkillers will do much to fight drug abuse," the *USA Today* editorial went on. "Only last year, *The Journal of the American Medical Association* published a study, based in part on the DEA's own data, concluding that increased pre-scribing of powerful painkillers did not increase drug abuse."

The study highlighted in the newspaper's editorial was the same one that David Haddox had been pointing other reporters toward ever since the OxyContin controversy started gaining national attention. At first glance, there seemed to be good reasons; for instance, the American Medical Association's publication, or *JAMA*, is considered one of this country's premier scientific journals.

The trouble was, however, that the study was irrelevant. It was based on hospital emergency room reports of prescription drug overdose cases reported into the Drug Abuse Warning Network, or DAWN, as the system is known. The system, which was underwritten by the federal government, had limited value because during the 1990s its data were often two or three years old when they were published. Also, its reporting hospitals were largely located in urban areas rather than in places like Lee County that were at the cutting edge of prescription narcotics abuse.

But most importantly, the *JAMA* study, though published in 2000, was based on an analysis of DAWN data from 1990 to 1996, a period of time that failed to reflect the subsequent surge in the prescribing of narcotics or even the introduction of Oxy-Contin. As a result, the report was already hopelessly outdated by the time it appeared.

In addition, the study's lead author, the University of Wisconsin's David Joranson had a long history of advocating increased narcotics use for pain patients. In a news release that accompanied the report's publication, Joranson and his colleagues celebrated the data as fulfilling their own prophecy that a wider medical use of narcotics wouldn't lead to increased abuse.

"This study suggests that increased use of opioid pain medications resulting in abuse may be based more on myth than reality," one of Joranson's coauthors wrote in 2000.

Now, however, some of the views championed by narcotics advocates were being dispelled even as the *JAMA* report appeared. Just a year or two after 1996, the cutoff date of Joranson's report, the number of emergency room reports involving prescription narcotics had started soaring. For instance, references to oxycodone-containing painkillers like OxyContin in DAWN reports between 1994 and 2001 climbed by 350 percent, far outpacing the growth rate of incidents involving hydrocodone-containing painkillers like Vicodin. In fact, by 2001 the total mentions of oxycodone-containing painkillers in DAWN reports were approaching those of hydrocodone-based drugs, even though those medications were prescribed three times as often.

As Purdue officials were contending with Laura Nagel, they also had to deal in the spring of 2001 with FDA officials and the future of OxyContin. Publicly they kept expressing concern that all the adverse publicity about the painkiller was stigmatizing pain patients. But the minutes of the first face-to-face meeting on April 23 between drug company and FDA officials suggest that Purdue executives had another concern—trying to convince the agency not to stigmatize OxyContin by singling it out for special attention.

A few months earlier, in December 2000, the company had sent a memo to its sales reps stating that it was "vital" for them to be forthright that the drug was being abused in some areas. At the same time, it added the phrase "when used properly for the management of pain" to the claim that OxyContin's slow-release formulation might lower its abuse appeal.

But it is clear from the minutes of the April 23 meeting that FDA officials had more extensive changes in mind about the claims Purdue would be permitted to make in the future for OxyContin. One involved the medical situations, or "indications," in agency jargon, in which the painkiller's use was recommended; another was the way the label delivered the drug's warnings.

According to the minutes of the April meeting, an FDA medical reviewer, Dr. Sharon Hertz, stated that

> The indication of "moderate to severe pain for patients who need to be on opiates for more than a few days" is broad and may not adequately reflect the intended population. The label should clearly state that this drug should be used only by patients who require opiates for an extended period of time, that it should not be utilized for first-time treatment of pain, and that it is not for intermittent use.

She further stated that a "black-box warning," the most severe warning the FDA can put on a medication, may be appropriate.

Another FDA official at the meeting, Dr. Cynthia G. McCormick, the director of the division of anesthetics, critical care, and addiction drug products, also questioned the value of some of the studies reviewed by the agency when it approved Oxy-Contin for some uses. And Dr. John K. Jenkins, director of the FDA's Office of Drug Evaluation, remarked that he believed OxyContin's label "will need a major overhaul."

Those Purdue executives at the meeting, who included Michael Friedman, Howard Udell, and David Haddox, didn't protest; they agreed to cooperate with the agency. But the FDA meeting notes make clear that they worried about any actions directed specifically at OxyContin. According to the FDA report:

> Purdue said they are having a difficult time understanding how abuse of OxyContin differs from abuse of other Schedule II drugs. They are concerned that they may create a perception that this drug is different. They would like to concur with the Agency's requests if the Agency will request the same of other companies. Dr. McCormick answered that there are sections of the label that are specific to OxyContin. The Agency will provide marked-up labeling when available. Dr. McCormick continued that if, by other companies, Purdue is referring to class labeling, that will take longer. The sponsor [Purdue] responded that they will address items specific or unique to OxyContin, but, for labeling issues that apply to all Schedule II drugs, they feel that the agency should make the request of others. They will not wait to make necessary changes, but feel that the request should be made to others. Dr. McCormick responded that the

immediate concern is OxyContin, particularly the
indication issue, and that other drugs will be addressed in
time. Dr. Hertz said that the general perception is that
OxyContin is not as potent as morphine. "More than a
few days" is not the same as "around the clock treatment
for an extended period of time after other drugs have
failed." Dental pain, for example, is a frivolous use of the
drug. Purdue concurred and added that Dr. Hertz'
description of the appropriate patient agrees with
perception of the appropriate patient for OxyContin.

One FDA official then inquired whether Purdue executives had
accurate data about the patient population using OxyContin.
Purdue responded that the only data it had were "anecdotal information."

In late July 2001, about four months after the negotiations between FDA and Purdue had begun, they finally reached a conclusion. The drugmaker and the agency announced a plan
under which Purdue would, among other things, drop the claim
that OxyContin's timed-release formulation had any relationship to a reduced risk of abuse. "Oxycodone can be abused in
a manner similar to other opioid agonists, legal or illicit," its
label now read. Purdue also agreed to put that information as
well as other dangers of the product in a black-box warning.

The plan also called for Purdue to revise the suggestion that
OxyContin be used to treat pain lasting "a few days or more"

by substituting the wording "for an extended period of time." The drugmaker also agreed to develop a plan to better detect OxyContin's abuse through such actions as receiving reports from drug treatment centers about the problems they were seeing with painkiller use.

Years later, one top FDA agency official admitted that the agency's actions reflected its acknowledgment that it had blundered when it approved claims for OxyContin back in 1995. "It clearly was being perceived as a severe problem when young, otherwise healthy people are dying and communities are having their people decimated," that official remembered. "We began to become acutely aware of how inaccurate the original label was and how it had probably contributed to the problem."

In July 2001, Purdue sent out an alert about the new warning and prescription information by overnight mail to eight hundred thousand doctors and pharmacists nationwide. In that letter, the company noted that it was "proud to be the first pharmaceutical manufacturer to voluntarily revise prescribing information" for a tightly controlled narcotic that addressed its abuse and diversion.

In a statement released by Purdue on that same day, Michael Friedman wrote: "Given the recent serious problems with abuse and diversion of the product in some areas of the country, the company believes that it is appropriate to make these changes at this time."

It certainly appeared to be an appropriate decision. But whether it was the appropriate time was another matter. By then, more than eight months had passed since Art Van Zee had met with David Haddox in November 2000 and urged the drugmaker to send out just such a warning.

Even as Purdue's letter went out, Laura Nagel was getting ready to send out one of her own. She still wasn't satisfied with the drugmaker's response and wanted to get to the bottom of the problem. By the summer of 2001, the diversion office had opened an investigation of Purdue's OxyContin plant in New Jersey because of reports that security at the facility was lax and that supplies of OxyContin were leaking out from it onto the street. She also decided to raise the stakes in her public battle with Purdue.

Nagel had told colleagues that nothing incensed her more than Purdue's apparent refusal to acknowledge its drug's role in overdose deaths. Nagel even shared with some of them a fantasy she had. In it, she brought Purdue executives to a darkened room and forced them to watch a slide show depicting every person who had died of an OxyContin-related overdose, along with a narration of his or her life. The drug company's executives would hear about the college student who had died of an overdose the first time he had tried OxyContin at a party. Then, they'd see a picture of a young teenage girl who had fatally overdosed.

Nagel knew from her experiences as a criminal agent that a certain number of drug overdose deaths were acceptable to society; few tears were spilled over dead junkies, and some people might even applaud the end of such lost and wasted lives. But she had come to believe that the toll being reaped by Oxy-Contin's misuse was unacceptable. The company was free to dispute the drug's role in every one of those deaths; in fact, it would be legal suicide for it to take any other position. Still, Nagel was determined to tally the death count as best she could.

That summer, medical examiners and coroners in more than thirty states received letters from the DEA asking them for highly specific information. Frederic Hellman, the county medical examiner south of Philadelphia, got one. So did William Massello, the state medical examiner in Virginia. The agency requested every medical examiner's report, autopsy report, and police report connected with any drug overdose death during the previous eighteen months in which oxycodone had turned up in the blood or bodily fluids of the dead.

Laura Nagel had launched her own counterattack; as far as she was concerned, the war wasn't over.

A TACIT UNDER-STANDING

IT TOOK A WHILE, BUT Sue Ella Kobak finally found a parking spot near the Lee County courthouse in Jonesville. She grabbed some legal files and began walking toward the redbrick building prepared for another day of frustrating work. Many of her cases now, in the summer of 2001, involved Oxy-Contin users who were in jail after breaking into homes or writing bad checks to get money to support their habit. Sue Ella expected to spend the next few hours going from one courtroom to the next, arguing with reluctant judges that her clients should go into drug treatment programs rather than prison. It usually didn't work.

On her way into the building this particular morning, she

noticed two men she didn't recognize. Strangers stuck out in Lee County, and Sue Ella knew everyone at the courthouse. Those she didn't know, for instance big-city lawyers from places like Richmond, she could spot by their dark business suits. But these men didn't fit that profile; both of them were wearing sports jackets and only one was wearing a tie.

At first she didn't think much about the pair. But as the day went on, she kept passing them in the hallway. On one occasion the men stared back at her as though they knew her. Sue Ella soon decided they probably worked for a real estate company and had come to the courthouse to check property title records. That afternoon, when she stopped by the county clerk's office, she found out the real reason. "Sue Ella," the clerk told her, "there have been two strangers here all day asking about you."

Sue Ella was bewildered. Then she assumed that the men had to be private investigators working for Purdue or one of its law firms who had come to Lee County to dig up dirt about her or Art. Another courthouse clerk called her the next morning to say that the men had ordered copies of various documents, including the title to Sue Ella's house and the file of an old court proceeding. They paid for the records with a $234 check made out from a small firm in Oakton, Virginia, a suburb of Washington, D.C. When Sue Ella searched the Internet for the company, she found its services were described as "business management consultants." She was tempted to call the company up and demand to know why it was snooping on her, but she decided instead to get a good laugh out of what the investigators had gotten for their $234.

It was the record of a decade-old case in which Sue Ella had been convicted of using "cursive and abusive language in public," a misdemeanor. At the time she had been working as the attorney for Lee County, handling all its corporate legal affairs, when a fellow county worker had written a letter sharply critical of how she had handled the buying of some law books. Sue Ella told the woman that she could take the letter and "stick it up your goddamn ass." Lawyers weren't supposed to use such phrases, and so Sue Ella was convicted and paid a $250 fine. Now, her sentiments were roughly similar as she thought about the two investigators reading through the case.

Sue Ella never learned why the investigators had come to Lee County, or who had hired them, but right around that same time Art Van Zee contacted a lawyer in Kentucky and agreed to testify in an OxyContin-related lawsuit. By mid-2001 a growing number of legal actions brought by plaintiffs' attorneys were claiming that Purdue and Abbott Laboratories, its marketing partner, should have to pay money to people who became addicted to OxyContin because the companies had failed to adequately warn of the drug's dangers. The West Virginia state attorney general, Darrell McGraw Jr., also sued both companies that same summer, contending that they had used "coercive and deceptive" techniques to market OxyContin. Both Purdue and Abbott denied the lawsuit allegations.

By now Van Zee had decided that lawsuits might achieve what the Lee Coalition's petition had failed to do—put a crimp in OxyContin's availability. Just a few months after it had been launched at Lee High, the petition was dead in the water; only about eighty-five hundred people ever signed it. Apart from some newspaper publicity, it had failed to generate much attention outside Lee County. Most lawmakers, regulators, and politicians on the state and federal levels supported Purdue's position that the drug needed to stay on the market. Meanwhile, the Internet site that Van Zee had created to publicize the recall effort had received a lot of negative messages.

"Are you a real doctor?" one person e-mailed Van Zee, according to a report in the *Roanoke Times*. "If you are, you should not be. I wouldn't send my dog to be treated by you."

However, the petition's failure hadn't dimmed Van Zee's resolve. Instead, as he continued to research the drug, his determination to do something about it only strengthened. A few months earlier, for instance, he had used an Internet service provided by the National Library of Medicine to track down the three research reports that narcotics proponents like Russell Portenoy had constantly cited when arguing for a wider use of narcotics, the reports that had served as the pain management movement's holy scientific trinity.

It took about a week for the reports to arrive by mail, but when Van Zee sat down to read them, he felt as though he had stepped through the looking glass. By no stretch of the imagination, he realized, did the studies show the kind of evidence for narcotics safety that pain management activists claimed they did. There was nothing in the reports, either individually or collectively, to suggest that the long-term risks to pain patients of abuse and addiction from narcotics like OxyContin were "less than one percent." In fact, the studies had nothing to do with the risks of the long-term use of narcotics for chronic pain.

That was just the beginning, though. As he read through the study about chronic sufferers, Van Zee could see that narcotics advocates had mischaracterized the report, either because they hadn't taken the trouble to read it or because they had decided to present data from the study in the light most favorable to their cause.

For example, some activists, such as Russell Portenoy, had been frequently quoted as saying that researchers looking at narcotics-related issues had found only "three problem cases among 2,369 patients" seen at the Diamond Headache Clinic in Chicago. But Van Zee could clearly see that depicting the study's statistics that way was misleading. While it was true that 2,369 headache sufferers had been admitted to the clinic during the eleven-month period when the study was conducted, researchers had looked at narcotics use in only a tiny subset of those patients: 62 people, to be precise. That group was made up of clinic patients who had taken either painkillers or a combination of painkillers and barbiturates for at least six months. Also, narcotics advocates never mentioned the report's conclusion, which didn't bode particularly well for their case. That 1977 finding: "There is a danger of dependency and abuse in patients with chronic headaches."

As it turned out, another report widely cited by narcotics

advocates—the one that found only four cases of drug-seeking behavior among 11,882 hospital patients who received various narcotics—wasn't even a scientific study. Instead, the data were contained in a 1980 letter submitted to the *New England Journal of Medicine* by Dr. Herschel Jick and Dr. Jane Porter of the Boston Collaborative Drug Surveillance Program, an initiative intended to help better identify dozens of prescription medication side effects.

In this case, pain management advocates had accurately characterized the data contained in the letter. But the problem was that the hospital statistics—which were the ones frequently extrapolated by narcotics activists to arrive at the 1 percent risk figure—were relevant to acute, or short-lived, pain rather than to the risks posed by the long-term use of narcotics for chronic pain. The reliability of the data was also called into question because drug abuse was simply one of the many side effects that the Boston Collaborative Drug Surveillance Program tried to monitor, and because patients weren't followed after they left the hospital.

A director of the project, Dr. Jick, would say years later that the statistics on narcotics and addiction had been sent to the *New England Journal of Medicine* as a letter because the data weren't adequate to be published as a study. He added that one couldn't conclude anything about the risks of long-term narcotics use from the figures. Jick recalled that prior to the start of the public debate over OxyContin, neither pain management activists nor drug companies such as Purdue had ever contacted him about the data. Then, once the controversy had started, people did start calling him, mainly plaintiffs' lawyers suing Purdue and defense attorneys defending the drugmaker.

It bothered Van Zee that narcotics advocates had used such half-baked science to popularize the widespread use of a powerful narcotic like OxyContin. Even now Purdue was continuing to paint the use and abuse of a drug like OxyContin in terms of black and white, with the black side being drug abusers and the white side being pain patients who somehow were protected from such pitfalls. But Van Zee was beginning to see that landscape for what it was: a murkier place of grays in which the painkiller's risks of addiction and abuse even for pain patients were greater than had been advertised.

In August 2001 the House of Representatives Energy and Commerce Committee's panel on Oversight and Investigations gathered for a hearing about OxyContin in a town meeting hall in Bensalem, Pennsylvania, a working-class suburb about twenty miles northeast of Philadelphia. Five months earlier, law enforcement officials there had arrested Dr. Richard G. Paolino and charged him with running a pill mill that dispensed Oxy-Contin and other prescription drugs. In coming months an increasing number of physicians would be arrested on similar charges, but Paolino's case was particularly noteworthy. Over a five-month period the Pennsylvania doctor, who wasn't a cancer or pain specialist, had written twelve hundred prescriptions for OxyContin, a rate of about ten a day. During Paolino's prescription-writing spree, five people around Bensalem, including four teenagers, had died in drug overdoses involving oxycodone, although he was not charged with any of those deaths.

The Bensalem hearing marked the first congressional inquiry into OxyContin, as well as the first opportunity for Purdue executives to testify under oath about what the company had done to respond to the drug's spreading abuse. It would also provide a public forum for the drugmaker to answer a crucial question that had hovered over the OxyContin controversy since its start: when had Purdue executives first learned about the drug's problems?

For company officials, the hearing was a critical watershed. Only a month had elapsed since the drugmaker had sent out its nationwide alert warning doctors about the painkiller's abuse, and Purdue was still under intense scrutiny. Sales of OxyContin had flattened amidst the controversy, and some states, seeing the expensive painkiller consume ever-growing chunks of their prescription drug spending, had begun requiring doctors, before prescribing it, to obtain special approval from officials charged with controlling medical expenditures.

At the Bensalem hearing, the congressmen first heard from a panel of law enforcement officials about Dr. Paolino's case. Then, Michael Friedman, Purdue's chief operating officer, took his place at the witness table. Behind him sat other Purdue executives including Howard Udell, Dr. Paul Goldenheim, a top company scientist, and Robin Hogen, the public relations head.

In a prepared statement, Friedman quickly addressed the question of when Purdue had first become aware of the painkiller's abuse. The company learned about the problem, said Friedman, in early 2000, at the same time and in the same manner as the public did—from reports in Maine newspapers. His statement continued: "Purdue immediately implemented a response team that included some of the company's top executives and scientists, including those who are here today. That team has committed Purdue to an unprecedented program to combat abuse and diversion."

Representative James C. Greenwood of Pennsylvania, the subcommittee's chairman, didn't press Friedman about why Purdue had relied on newspapers to monitor its drug's abuse. Instead, he started to question him about another interesting issue. Greenwood was curious about why Purdue hadn't taken measures to crack down on Dr. Paolino, since the company could see that his prescribing volume was way out of line based on the data it purchased from IMS Health, the company that collected prescription data from pharmacies.

"When you see a doctor who is not associated with Fox Chase Cancer Center but is a little osteopath here in Bensalem, doing this vast number," Greenwood asked Friedman, "what do you do with that information?"

Initially Friedman, while testifying for the first time in such a high-pressure setting, seemed confident in his answers, as though repeating well-rehearsed lines.

"We have learned over the years," he replied, "that the absolute number of prescriptions that a physician is prescribing is, in and of itself, not an indicator of the doctor doing something wrong. We don't measure or assess how well a doctor practices medicine. We are not in the office with a physician and a patient observing the examination or involved in that process. We know, for example, . . ."

Greenwood cut off the Purdue executive and began pressing him about the IMS data.

"Why do you want that information then?"

"Well, we use that information to understand what is happening in terms of the development of use of our product in any area," Friedman responded.

"You want to see how successful your marketing techniques are?" Greenwood asked.

"Sure," Friedman replied, as he began to look uncomfortable and started glancing around at his Purdue colleagues for support.

After some more questions, Greenwood got to his point. He challenged Friedman to explain why Purdue used IMS data to measure its marketing success but not to monitor whether doctors were properly prescribing OxyContin. "That is the other side of your responsibility," he told Friedman. "Why wouldn't you have been using this data to make sure that the Dr. Paolinos of the world weren't wrecking the reputation of your product?"

It was right around then that Howard Udell leaned forward and started whispering to Friedman. It was apparently decided to let the company's top lawyer do its talking.

"I think Mr. Udell might be able to respond to that more," Friedman told Greenwood.

Udell insisted that Purdue couldn't have known from the

178

IMS data alone that Paolino was a renegade physician. And he added that law enforcement officials were far better suited than a drugmaker like Purdue to investigate problem doctors.

Greenwood didn't appear satisfied with that. "It seems to me that your company has a responsibility to be looking at this data and not relying on what law enforcement tells you. . . . And I don't understand why that hasn't been something that you have been aggressively doing."

For Purdue, there was little to be gained from getting into an argument with Greenwood. So Udell found a graceful way out.

"I think we learned a lot from the case of Dr. Paolino," he told the official. "The picture that is painted in the newspaper is of a horrible, bad actor, someone who preyed on this community, who caused untold suffering. And he fooled us all. He fooled law enforcement. He fooled the DEA. He fooled local law enforcement. He fooled us."

At the start of 2001, Lindsay Myers had done a good job fooling her parents that her methadone treatment was going well. Then, just after Mother's Day that year, Johnny's wallet disappeared.

Jane had gotten a Dustbuster as a present and Ray offered to put up a bracket in the kitchen closet so she could hang it there. Johnny always put his shoes in that same closet when he came in from work and stuck his wallet inside one of them for safekeeping. But when he got up to get his shoes after Ray and Lindsay were done in the kitchen hanging up the Dustbuster his wallet was missing.

Jane called over to Ray's house and told Lindsay to get back home. When Lindsay and Ray arrived, Johnny demanded to know if either one of them had taken the wallet. They both denied it. That's when Jane told Lindsay that she was bringing her down to Lee County hospital for a drug test.

It was fine with Lindsay, she said; she didn't have anything to hide. So she and Ray got into the Mercedes and Jane started down the hill toward the hospital. A month earlier, Jane and Lindsay had been through the same exercise. At that time, Lindsay had broken down just as they passed the mailbox at the bottom of the hill and confessed that she had been dabbling a little with drugs again. This time as they drove past the mailbox Lindsay didn't say a word. Jane took that as a good sign; maybe everything was okay, and she started to relax.

Lindsay was equally at ease inside the hospital's emergency room as they waited for her drug screen to come back. Finally, an emergency room doctor appeared and told Jane that Lindsay had tested positive for cocaine. Jane was stunned and Ray shot a glance at Lindsay. None of them talked on the ride back from the hospital, and after Jane parked the Mercedes in the garage she stayed inside the car while Lindsay drove Ray home. In the meantime, Jane just sat there and cried.

When Lindsay returned, she got into the car with Jane. Lindsay said that she really wasn't doing drugs again; it was just that she had run into a boy she knew who had some cocaine.

She swore that she would have told her mother all about it if Ray hadn't been there but he was so jealous he would have gone crazy.

She leaned over toward her mother and told her that this time she really needed her help. "Please don't tell him anything, Mom," Lindsay said. "If he finds out about this he might break up with me."

In January 2002, a meeting with significant consequences for the future regulation of narcotics, including OxyContin, took place. At that time, a special advisory panel to the FDA gathered to propose changes to how the agency oversees and manages existing narcotics stocks and approves new opioid-containing drugs.

Both that FDA meeting and other congressional hearings had been originally scheduled to follow on the heels of the Bensalem hearing the previous August. But just two weeks afterward, the cataclysmic events of September 11 focused the country's attention on more vital threats.

The panel's two days of public meetings took place in the ballroom of a Holiday Inn in Gaithersburg, Maryland, the Washington suburb where the FDA is located. Members of the panel included such pain management luminaries as Kathleen Foley of Memorial Sloan-Kettering. Russell Portenoy was also there, serving as a consultant to the group. About 150 people, many of them drug company officials, attended the sessions. Representatives of pain care advocacy groups showed up in force, and Art Van Zee made the eight-hour drive from Lee County to take part in the gathering.

The FDA panel was headed by Dr. Nathaniel Paul Katz, who had served as director of the pain center at Brigham and Women's Hospital in Boston. The short, boyish-looking Katz, who was thirty-nine at the time, was an interesting choice to lead the panel, because while he believed in the medical value of long-acting narcotics like OxyContin, he had never championed their widespread use. He was a researcher and had long known what Art Van Zee had only recently learned: that the reports used to suggest a minute risk from long-term narcotics use were scientifically worthless. He also believed there was a similar dearth of research in another critical area; it wasn't at all clear which pain patients benefited best from drugs like Oxy-Contin, or for how long the medication's positive effects outweighed its negative ones.

Before the meeting, FDA officials had told Katz that they didn't want the panel's public sessions to degenerate into a debate over OxyContin, and he sounded that message in his opening remarks.

"The goal of this meeting is not to take any particular drugs off the market," Katz emphasized. "It's not to focus on any specific drugs. We're trying to deal with the opioids as a class, since they all share very similar properties, not to focus on any particular members of that class."

OxyContin, however, wouldn't be kept out of the room. In their comments to the panel, a procession of pain patients, nurses, and narcotics advocates all expressed their concerns that the FDA not take any actions that would restrict the availability of OxyContin and similar drugs.

"On several occasions we have had people who were literally threatening suicide as they were speaking to us," said John Giglio, the executive director of one advocacy group, the American Pain Foundation. "Unfortunately, most of the media reports fail to convey the other side of the story, that millions of people suffer from serious chronic pain; yet most go untreated or undertreated, especially the elderly, minorities, the poor, and children."

The day's most eagerly awaited speaker was Russell Portenoy. Panel members had asked him to give a talk that would put into perspective the difficult issues with which they were grappling.

As Portenoy began his talk, Nathaniel Katz leaned back to listen. Katz was only a decade younger than Portenoy, but like many other physicians in the room he viewed the physician as an inspirational figure, the elder statesman of the pain management movement.

Portenoy recounted the long history of inadequate pain care and the biases against narcotics that had existed once among pain experts. He then described with pride the subsequent sea change that led to the drugs' greater use, and how pain patients had benefited. That dramatic turnabout wouldn't have happened, Portenoy said, without the support of both the pharmaceutical industry and the news media, which had been extremely sympathetic to the plight of pain patients.

But then he suddenly shifted gears. It was now clear to him

that both pain management activists and drugmakers, fearful of a backlash, had failed to openly and adequately address the potential of narcotics to produce abuse and addiction.

As he put it, there'd been "a tacit reluctance on the part of supporters, including pain specialists, those in the media who have been portraying the problem of undertreatment, patient advocates and industry to discuss the legitimate risk associated with opioid toxicity and abuse addiction because of the concern that if we opened up Pandora's box and talked about addiction and abuse, all of the progress that had been made during the past ten years would be lost."

Then, he added, "There has been a bit of a tacit understanding that we won't talk about it too much. We do need to talk about it."

Even as he championed the value of narcotics, Portenoy now added his voice to those like Art Van Zee who had been arguing that too many doctors were too freely prescribing powerful painkillers even though they didn't have the time or the proper training to assess or monitor their patients for drug abuse.

"Generalists are adopting the therapy without adequate knowledge of pain management principles," he said. "This we already knew, but also without adequate knowledge of opioid pharmacology and addiction medicine principles and thereby perhaps placing patients at risk for the adverse effects of opioid drugs in this broad phenomenon of chemical dependency that wouldn't be there if the clinicians had better skills and training in addiction medicine principles."

Once his talk was done, Portenoy answered questions from the panel's members. In responding to one, he reiterated his belief that doctors shouldn't be prescribing powerful narcotics if they didn't have basic training in how to do so safely.

"If you don't have it, don't do it," he said. "Don't prescribe."

Nathaniel Katz almost fell out of his chair. Not only had Portenoy's speech struck him as a mea culpa, but he was impressed that Portenoy had given it before an audience of drug company officials who had underwritten his research. Art Van Zee, who had been the lone voice that day arguing for a tightening of FDA rules, had also been riveted. When the hearing ended, he spotted Portenoy and Kathleen Foley standing together in the hotel's lobby and asked to meet with them. They agreed to do so before the start of the following day's session.

The next morning when Van Zee returned to the hotel's lobby, Portenoy was alone and explained that Kathleen Foley was running a little late. Van Zee told Portenoy that he had been absorbed by his speech because it had zeroed in on some of his own concerns. He asked the Mt. Sinai expert what he thought was an acceptable level of risk from the drugs given that it was clear that the 1 percent figure was meaningless.

"If it is 1 percent and you have ten million people on opioids, that's one thing," Van Zee said. "But what if it is 5 percent or 6 percent? What do you consider acceptable collateral damage? If you create fifty thousand patients that are opioid addicts?"

Later, Russell Portenoy would say that he had never sought

to miscast the earlier reports or their meaning. The claims made for those studies, he insisted, were really an artifact of their time; Portenoy would say that so little was known in the late 1980s and early 1990s about the risk of long-term narcotics use that both supporters and opponents of the drugs alike simply grabbed at whatever data were out there.

That day in early 2002, however, Portenoy was miffed by Van Zee's comments, finding them extreme. Portenoy believed that even if the risk were 5 percent, that meant that 95 percent of people with severe pain could safely use a drug like Oxy-Contin without concern, a number he considered remarkable.

Portenoy and Van Zee were equally well intentioned. It was just that their differing perspectives on OxyContin had shaped their very different views. Portenoy's talk on the painkiller reflected his position on the front line of dealing with the most intractable cases of pain, while Van Zee saw the drug from a very different perspective; in places like Lee County its easy accessibility and its abuse seemed to go hand in hand. They might have stood there all day arguing without agreeing with each other.

Just then, however, Kathleen Foley appeared. In recent years Foley's already vaunted medical reputation had risen further as a result of her efforts to improve the pain care of the dying. She mentioned to Van Zee that she had just seen a television documentary about OxyContin abuse. Foley said that she had been deeply distressed by the scenes of addicted kids shown on the program, and she urged Van Zee to think about compiling his data about OxyContin so he could get it published.

She then offered him another perspective on Purdue. "You should understand about Purdue," she said to him. "There are people who have been in pain management for a long time and who have seen a lot that Purdue has done in this field—not only in making medicines available to people who can't pay, but they've seen real improvements in pain management."

Foley spoke about the company's educational role and the hundreds of seminars it had sponsored to help doctors better understand pain. Van Zee wasn't swayed. "I really think they are more promotional than educational," he said.

Foley, who was close to the Sackler family, bristled at his comments and excused herself. Portenoy also walked away. In the space of ten minutes, Van Zee had managed to exasperate them both.

After its deliberations, however, the FDA advisory panel made recommendations that rang a chord with Van Zee. The group urged that the agency adopt guidelines requiring that a narcotic manufacturer seeking to get a new drug approved first develop a program that would closely monitor its abuse and addiction as soon as it went onto the market. The panel also suggested that drug producers be required to undertake tests aimed at determining the effectiveness of narcotics over longer periods of time.

Even before Russell Portenoy's appearance before the FDA panel, some pain management activists had begun to feel the ground shift under their feet as a result of OxyContin. While they continued to bash the media for what they saw as their excesses in reporting about the painkiller's abuse, a few experts also acknowledged that they had helped set the OxyContin problem into motion by downplaying the risks of narcotics and overstating the abuse resistance of longer-acting drugs.

For example, Dr. Steven D. Passik, a pain management expert and Purdue consultant who had also served on the FDA advisory panel, had issued his own mea culpa in a letter that was published in the *Journal of Pain and Symptom Management* in May 2001.

Recently there have been two rather inflammatory and cynical sounding articles in *Time* and *Forbes* about the abuse and diversion of controlled-release oxycodone (OxyContin) as an emerging problem in pain management. This issue concerns everyone involved in pain management and we should be able to respond to patients, the media, and regulators. This is not Purdue Pharma's problem; the abuse of an opioid commonly used in pain management is a sensitive topic and requires reasoned responses from experts.

Unfortunately, the problem of opioid abuse during the course of pain management is an issue over which—I'm afraid—those of us in the pain management community have been somewhat disingenuous. While I certainly believe that the risk of addiction, abuse and poor adherence (aberrant drug-related behavior) in the use of these medications is far less than was once believed to be the case, it is not zero. In our zeal to improve access to opioids and relieve patient suffering, pain specialists have understated the problem, drawing faulty conclusions from very limited data. In effect, we have told primary care doctors and other prescribers that the risk was so low that they essentially could ignore the possibility of addiction. We have also overstated the concept that long-acting drugs have a lower risk of abuse.

The data which have been used to justify this position are derived from cancer patients treated in [specialized] care centers (who have a low base rate of addiction and, therefore, are not representative of the population as a whole), clinical trial subject to selection biases and limited survey data. For example, the oft-cited Porter and Jick study was a study of acute, not chronic, pain; a less than 1% risk of addiction among non-addicts in an acute care setting does not define the risk to the diverse chronic pain population during long-term exposure. Moreover, it represents one end of the continuum—the other end would be long-term opioid treatment for pain in an addict population. At this end of the continuum, we have very limited data; in a small number of patients, the risk of aberrant drug behavior was 45%.

Doctors must be taught to assess where a given patient falls along this continuum of addiction risk. Further, doctors must assess a patient's psychosocial condition, situation and subculture well enough to judge the risk of diversion.

Six years earlier, on the eve of OxyContin's launch, those precise sentiments had been sounded by a few experts like Dennis Turk, the clinical psychologist. Turk's cautions as well as others issued during the intervening years had gone unheeded. But now the OxyContin crisis had started to change that. Even Purdue, which for years had promoted the painkiller to doctors by repeatedly citing data from that same Porter and Jick study, had begun to back away from earlier pronouncements.

For example, at a meeting in April 2002 of the American Society of Addiction Medicine, a professional group that represents drug abuse treatment specialists, Dr. Sidney H. Schnoll, a drug abuse expert who had recently been hired by Purdue, was asked to estimate the addiction risks posed by long-term narcotics use. Schnoll gave the one reply that couldn't be challenged; he said he had "no idea."

The management of Purdue, after selling more than $2 billion of OxyContin, had apparently come to the same conclusion. Since early 1996 it had emphatically told doctors that "iatrogenic 'addiction' to opioids legitimately used in the management of pain is very rare." One company-sponsored training program for doctors had even called it "exquisitely rare." But by the time of Dr. Schnoll's appearance at the American Society of Addiction Medicine's conference in 2002, the company had changed its tune. Now it was using a new package insert to tell both doctors prescribing OxyContin and patients getting the drug, "We do not know how often patients with continuing (chronic) pain become addicted to narcotics, but the risk has been reported to be small."

It was also at that same conference in Atlanta that Art Van Zee and Nathaniel Katz, the FDA panel's chairman, ran into each other. Katz had come to give a talk. Van Zee was there because he had realized that to do his job right he needed fresh training. The FDA had recently announced plans to approve a new methadone substitute for drug addicts called buprenorphine. Previously, people seeking addiction treatment had to go to methadone clinics. Buprenorphine, however, was intended to be prescribed by doctors because experts believed that more drug abusers would seek help if they could get it in the privacy of a physician's office.

To prescribe the most powerful narcotics, a doctor just filled out the paperwork needed to get a DEA license. But to treat people who had become addicted to such drugs, the FDA was requiring that doctors get certified to use buprenorphine by going through a training course that lasted several hours. Van Zee had come to the Atlanta meeting to attend such a session.

While he was there he heard Katz's talk and later went up to speak with him. He explained to the pain specialist that he had been spending months looking for more studies that had addressed the abuse risks to patients of long-term narcotics use. Katz looked at Van Zee and smiled.

"There's a reason you didn't find any," he told him. "They don't exist."

Van Zee walked away shaking his head; for years, he realized, medicine had been flying blind.

THE SECRETS OF DENDUR

NEARLY FOUR DECADES before a congressional subcommittee questioned Purdue executives in Bensalem, Pennsylvania, about OxyContin, Dr. Arthur M. Sackler, the founder of his family's pharmaceutical dynasty, testified before another congressional committee, this one in the Senate. As fate would have it, the senators in 1962 were looking into whether pharmaceutical companies were promoting drugs using misleading claims or tactics.

At the time, the advertising and marketing of prescription drugs directly to doctors was a relatively new industry practice. But already by the early 1960s, concerns about the proliferation of misleading and deceptive drug advertisements were pervasive, prompting the investigation by a Senate Judiciary Committee subcommittee.

It was little wonder that Arthur Sackler had been called to testify. At the time, he headed the country's largest advertising agency devoted to the marketing of pharmaceuticals, William Douglas McAdams in New York City. But the agency was only the most visible symbol of Sackler's dominance of the promotional end of the drug industry. His web of business interests was so vast and complex that details about its influential extent emerged only after his death in 1987 at the age of seventy-three.

Arthur Sackler was a complex person of extraordinary will and determination, lionized by his friends and admirers as a Renaissance man with a passion for science and a boundless entrepreneurial vision. He was a visionary whose vast energies allowed him to pursue multiple careers simultaneously. As a medical student he also worked as a drug-advertising copywriter, and for a time he was both a research psychiatrist and a top pharmaceutical marketing executive.

Starting in the 1940s, Sackler created a sprawling drug industry octopus whose tentacles reached into every aspect of how drugs were made, marketed, advertised, and sold. While his agency created advertisements and promotional campaigns for prescription drugs, Sackler consulted with some of the world's biggest drug companies, helping them define the medical conditions for which their medications should be marketed as cures. He also controlled a chain of scientific journals that carried research articles about new drugs—drugs produced by his advertising clients. And Sackler also created less obvious, though no less effective, outlets for his clients to reach both doctors and the ultimate consumers of drugs: the public. For instance, the editorial tone of the *Medical Tribune*, a bi-weekly newspaper that Sackler distributed for free to about 168,000 doctors nationwide, often echoed the editorial views of the drugmakers that advertised in it. Meanwhile, various firms controlled by Arthur Sackler created and distributed "articles" to newspapers that were really marketing plugs for the drug companies that paid for them. In doing so, Sackler presided over the birth of the "infomercial," a means of pharmaceutical promotion that, in time, would become ubiquitous. Such planted stories were also the forerunners of the classic problem/solution marketing strategy, later proposed by Purdue officials, in which a "survey" spotlighting the inadequate treatment of pain was to have been distributed to newspapers and publications to boost OxyContin sales.

In his 1962 Senate appearance, Arthur Sackler frequently faced hostile questioning, some from a formidable adversary, legendary senator Estes Kefauver, the Tennessee Democrat who had unsuccessfully run for vice president on Adlai Stevenson's 1956 presidential ticket. At one point Kefauver asked Sackler about a small public relations company called Medical and Science Communications Associates, a firm that distributed "news" articles that were actually drug-company marketing tools.

Sackler acknowledged to the senators that William Douglas McAdams had worked with Medical and Science Communications. But Sackler adamantly denied that he had any influence over the public relations firm's activities even though the firm happened to be located at the same address as his agency, on Lexington Avenue. "I never had any stock in Medical and Science Communications, and I was never an officer," Sackler avowed.

Strictly speaking, his sworn testimony was correct. The corporate paperwork did not list him as either a company officer or a shareholder. But in fact, the company's sole shareholder was Else Sackler, the doctor's then-wife, the first of three. Over the years it was common practice for Sackler to put the names of his wives, children, or business associates on corporate documents.

Sackler walked away unscathed from the Senate hearing, his reputation unblemished. He had handled himself magnificently, referring frequently to his extensive medical credentials—his directorship of a psychiatric research facility, his publication of sixty scientific papers, and his memberships in prestigious organizations such as the New York Academy of Sciences—as proof that the advertisements created by his agency were based on science and not hyperbole. While quietly displaying his contempt for bureaucrats and lawmakers, he had managed to keep the details of his business dealings private. Like the marketing genius he was, Arthur Sackler had created an illusion and disappeared.

Operating in secrecy was the preference of all three Sackler brothers who founded Purdue, but that was especially true for

Arthur, the undisputed head of the family. He was a man who lived by only one guiding star and played by only one set of rules—his own.

Irrespective of the names on corporate documents or letterhead, Arthur controlled everything in his realm, even at times his brothers, Mortimer and Raymond. "In my mind, it was all Arthur," said Win Gerson, a top executive at William Douglas McAdams, explaining Sackler's business dealings to a lawyer after his death. "I guess legally you had to break it out into different, quote, affiliated companies, and these are the legal entities. But actually to me the whole thing was Arthur."

Sackler spent the last years of his life using the massive fortune he had earned to acquire world-renowned collections of Asian antiquities, European bronzes, and exquisite majolica ceramics. He counted Linus Pauling, the Nobel Prize-winning chemist, among his friends. He talked art and politics with Anwar as-Sadat, the president of Egypt, and Moshe Dayan, the Israeli defense minister. And he socialized with some of the cultural and social lights of his day, from painter Marc Chagall to sculptor Isamu Noguchi to opera singer Richard Tucker.

Today, Arthur Sackler's name adorns museums, medical schools, and other institutions worldwide. Along with his younger brothers, he financed the construction of the Sackler Wing at the Metropolitan Museum of Art in New York City. A striking glass-curtained structure, it houses treasures from the age of the Egyptian pharaohs, most notably the Temple of Dendur, a stone shrine that is the Sackler Wing's centerpiece.

There is the Arthur M. Sackler Gallery at the Smithsonian Institution in Washington, D.C., the Arthur M. Sackler Museum at Harvard University in Massachusetts, and the Arthur M. Sackler Museum of Art and Archaeology at Beijing University in China.

All of his giving gained Arthur Sackler entry to a tier of society far above his humble origins. The son of Jewish immigrants from Eastern Europe, he was born and grew up in the Flatbush section of Brooklyn, New York, then a working-class neighborhood. His father's business failed during the Depression and he later opened a small grocery store. To help his family financially, Arthur got his first taste of advertising, selling ads for local newspapers and other publications. He graduated from New York University in 1933 and went on to get his medical degree from the same school.

From the beginning, he comfortably juggled different careers. The year 1944, for example, was a big one for the young doctor. He became both president of William Douglas McAdams and a psychiatric resident at Creedmoor State Hospital in Queens, New York. And those dual duties did not seem to slow him down. Even as his advertising business flourished, Arthur rose through the ranks at Creedmoor, a hospital for the mentally ill, and eventually became director of a research center there called the Institute for Psychobiologic Studies.

If not for the financial lures of business, Arthur Sackler might have gone on to an important career as a research scientist. He played a prominent role in early efforts to understand the chemistry of mental illness. In the early 1950s, he and some associates at Creedmoor published numerous papers that suggested the blood chemistry of schizophrenics was different from that of emotionally healthy people. They also attempted to develop blood tests that would serve as screening devices to identify those suffering from serious mental illness.

But by the early 1950s, Sackler was already wealthy; he was making so much money in business that he was subsidizing the Creedmoor research institute he directed. And while Arthur's direct involvement with scientific research would slacken, his impact on the pharmaceutical industry became massive and enduring. Simply put, Sackler was the godfather of the modern-day drug advertising industry. Many of the marketing and promotional techniques still used fifty years later by pharmaceutical producers were invented or refined by him.

At one time, for instance, drug companies didn't directly advertise prescription drugs to doctors, and certainly not in medical publications. But all that changed after World War II with the rapid development of the American pharmaceutical industry and Arthur Sackler's appearance on the scene.

Beginning in the late 1940s and early 1950s, drugmakers began not only to greatly expand the types of medications they produced but also to shorten the life span of each drug they manufactured to make way for "new" or "improved" versions. It was the era of the "wonder" drug, as waves of new antibiotics, tranquilizers, psychotropic drugs, and other medications burst out from the pharmaceutical industry, each offering the hope that it could cure an illness or a condition once thought resistant to treatment.

Previously, sales reps were the ones who introduced physicians to a new medication produced by their company. But in 1952, Arthur Sackler engineered a watershed event that would change the interaction between pharmaceutical makers and physicians forever. That year, a multipage color insert produced for Pfizer Laboratories by William Douglas McAdams for its antibiotic Terramycin appeared in an issue of the *Journal of the American Medical Association*. From that point forward, the financial entanglements between drugmakers and doctors would only increase.

Arthur Sackler believed that drug advertising, marketing, and promotion all played a vital role in keeping physicians current with the pharmaceutical industry's rapidly changing landscape of products. In an interview in the 1950s with the publication *Advertising Age*, Sackler remarked that only about 20 percent of the money pharmaceutical makers directed toward drug advertising was spent on direct brand promotion. Instead, the vast bulk of such funds, he explained, was used for physician "education."

"The bulk of money being spent [on advertising] is primarily for informational and educational uses," Sackler was quoted by *Advertising Age* as saying. "The term 'advertising budget' is therefore a misnomer. This 'promotion' is as essential for the safe and proper use of drugs as good driving and accident prevention campaigns are for the safe and proper use of automobiles."

Under the rubric of physician "education," Sackler breathed

life into another arm of the drug marketing industry that would soon spring up. Within a few years, virtually every pharmaceutical company was sponsoring so-called continuing medical education courses for health professionals, or CMEs, essentially hour-long talks about medical issues that also served as vehicles to pitch or promote its drugs. And decades later, Purdue would spend a small fortune flying in physicians to conferences about inadequate treatment of pain and the need for doctors to aggressively use long-acting narcotics like OxyContin in pain's treatment.

But Arthur Sackler not only paved new ways for marketing drugs, he helped create a new chapter in American life—the emergence of the pill as a quick fix. The feel-good tranquilizers of the 1960s, Librium and Valium, were immortalized in Jacquelin Susann's novel *The Valley of the Dolls*, and the Rolling Stones's hit song "Mother's Little Helper." However, it was Arthur Sackler's marketing genius that turned Librium and Valium into not only the greatest pharmaceutical successes of their era but also medicine chest and nightstand drawer staples throughout the United States.

Pharmacologically, Librium and Valium belonged to the same class of drugs, the benzodiazepines; they worked similarly to calm a patient's nerves, and both were potentially addicting. But Arthur, working as a consultant to the drugs' producer, Hoffman-LaRoche of Switzerland, skillfully promoted them as though they were two entirely different medications so that doctors would use them for different problems and the two products would not cannibalize each other's sales. He positioned Librium, which was launched first, as a treatment for "anxiety" while promoting Valium for a separate set of mental concerns and preoccupations that he defined as "psychic tension."

Using that battle plan, Roche Labs, Hoffman-LaRoche's subsidiary in the United States, spent between $150 million and $200 million during the 1960s to promote its twin tranquilizers, a level of spending never before seen in the pharmaceutical industry. As John Pekkanen wrote in his 1973 book *The American Connection*, that money was used to unleash an unprecedented promotional campaign for Librium and Valium aimed at both doctors and the public.

> The whole drug industry campaign for mood drugs in the
> 1960s was to broaden to absurd limits the definition of
> *illness* to include every upset, every disappointment, and
> every vague problem encountered in day-to-day living.
> Each was a ripe candidate for drug-taking. If the facts in
> these ads were not untruths, then their implications often
> were. Roche Labs pushed its tranquilizer twins for a
> variety of "illnesses," although they were careful never to
> urge the use of Librium and Valium for treatment of the
> same problem. But the cumulative effect of the advertising
> in medical journals was to cover every problem
> encountered in a doctor's office: tension, anxiety, muscle
> spasms, even something called the "intervals," described
> as that worrisome time when one wonders about some

dark possibility in the future. Rapid pulse, faintness, breathlessness, missed periods, hot flashes, fear, and depression were all apt candidates for either tranquilizers, stimulants, depressants, or antidepressants, or all of those. There was a chemical solution for everything.

Arthur Sackler, already a rich man, made an emperor's fortune from Librium and Valium. Under the terms of his agreement with Hoffman-LaRoche, he received bonus payments based on the volume of pills sold. The Swiss drugmaker was so grateful to Sackler that it provided him with millions of dollars in interest-free loans as advances against future advertising work, money that he quickly invested to make yet another fortune in the stock market.

But while many saw Arthur Sackler's career as the rise of a self-made man, others viewed him far differently, as a relentless and sometimes ruthless competitor who often cloaked his pursuit of profit and power behind the veil of science and research. In creating the modern-day pharmaceutical advertising industry, he also helped pioneer some of its most controversial and misleading practices: the showering of favors on doctors, the lavish spending on consultants and experts ever ready to back a drugmaker's claims, the funding of supposedly independent medical interest groups, the creation of publications that serve as industry mouthpieces, or the outright expropriation of scientific research for promotional purposes.

The promotional gimmicks used by his advertising firms often smacked less of high-minded science than of the handicraft of a huckster working the frontiers of a wild and untamed industry. For instance, one medical brochure produced by Sackler's advertising firm for Pfizer Laboratories promoting an antibiotic called Sigmamycin depicted business cards of physicians in various cities as though they were testimonials to the drug's effectiveness. The cards were extremely realistic looking, containing details such as each physician's address, telephone number, and even office hours. But when a curious journalist once tried to contact the doctors cited in the ad, he found out that they didn't exist.

The work of real doctors and scientists could also serve as putty to be reshaped by the skilled hands of the admen working for Arthur Sackler. In the 1950s, for instance, an ad announcing the discovery of a "happy baby vitamin" appeared in a free weekly newsletter produced by William Douglas McAdams and distributed to doctors on behalf of the Upjohn Company, a major drugmaker. That vitamin, pyridoxine or B_6, also happened to be contained in an Upjohn product, Zymabasic drops. The advertisement, depicting a sleep-deprived father holding an infant, read:

> The wakeful baby who turns father into a floor walker may simply lack B_6. Infants formula and mother's milk frequently fail to provide sufficient amounts of this "happy baby vitamin." That's why basic baby supplementation calls for Zymabasic, the formula with all four: A, D, and C, plus B_6.

But in 1958, Dr. Charles B. May, the editor of *Pediatrics*, the medical journal of the American Academy of Pediatrics, decided to investigate. Alarmed by the sudden appearance of a bevy of infant supplements containing B_6, he contacted several scientists to determine whether Upjohn and other drugmakers were appropriately using their research in advertisements. "I would appreciate your letting me know if you believe your work had been properly exploited by those who urge its universal use as a supplement to the infant's diet," May wrote in July 1958 to those researchers. Their reaction was uniform; for example, Arild E. Hansen of the University of Texas quickly replied that his work on B_6's effect on colicky babies was so preliminary and inconclusive that he had dropped it. "Never by any stretch of the imagination have we inferred that there is such a thing as a 'happy baby vitamin'," Dr. Hansen wrote. He and the other scientists all said that they had never been informed by drugmakers that their research was being cited in product promotions. More than four decades later, Dr. Herschel Jick of the Boston Collaborative Drug Surveillance Program would find himself in much the same situation with respect to OxyContin.

As the powerful lord of his realm, Arthur Sackler didn't hesitate to make careers or crush them, inspiring not only intense loyalty among his employees and business associates, but also terror. In addition, he used his vast empire of publications both to promote uncritically the interests of his friends and corporate allies and to savage and seek to destroy those who stood in his way.

One favored vehicle was the *Medical Tribune*, the newspaper that Sackler distributed to 168,000 doctors nationwide. He used the publication as a platform for his personal philosophies and political views. The column he wrote called "One Man and Medicine" regularly disparaged regulators as overreaching, sang the praises of unbridled scientific research, and occasionally took potshots at other industries. For example, he hated cigarettes and also lambasted automakers for failing to quickly install seat belts. Arthur also used the *Medical Tribune* like a mother goose to protect the golden eggs of his drug industry advertisers, particularly the big pharmaceutical companies that produced brand-name prescription medications.

Apart from government, there may have been no greater enemy for Sackler and his clients than manufacturers of "generic" drugs who quickly knocked off cheaper-selling versions of proprietary medications such as Purdue's MS Contin once their patents had expired. Arthur contended that generic drugs were not necessarily equal in effectiveness to their more expensive brand-name rivals, and the *Medical Tribune* published news articles about generics that depicted them as the pharmaceutical equivalent of a Red menace.

For instance, one *Medical Tribune* article was entitled "Schizophrenics 'Wild' on Weak Generic," according to an account in the *New York Times*. In it, Sackler's publication described how "all hell broke loose" at a Veterans Administration hospital after patients on its psychiatric intensive care floor were switched from the brand-name antipsychotic drug Thorazine to a generic equivalent. The article went on to relate how eleven previously stabilized patients had run amok until they were switched back to Thorazine, and how their behavior returned to normal "as if a switch had been flipped."

The FDA investigated the episode and its officials found that the report cited in the *Medical Tribune* and its claim against the generic were so scientifically flawed as to be useless.

As he rose through the pharmaceutical industry and the ranks of society transforming everything he touched, Arthur Sackler also shaped the careers and destinies of his brothers. Arthur was only three years older than Mortimer and seven years older than Raymond. But he treated them not as siblings but more like his progeny and understudies. He got them into medical schools and paid for their training as research psychiatrists. He got them jobs at Creedmoor Institute for Psychobiologic Studies, the research facility he funded. And after Mortimer and Raymond were fired in 1953 from Creedmoor after refusing to sign a McCarthy-era loyalty oath, Arthur stepped in again, setting up his brothers in the business of making drugs.

Mortimer and Raymond Sackler were highly intelligent and accomplished men who, like their older brother, would give generously to the arts, science, and medicine. But they were also part of the world of Arthur Sackler and spent part of their lives working in his shadow. Dr. Stanley Graham, a psychiatrist in New York who worked in the early 1950s at the Creedmoor

Institute, recalled years later how Arthur treated his brothers like the rest of the hired help whenever he visited the facility.

"He told everyone exactly what to do, including Morty and Ray," Graham remembered.

By taking care of his brothers, Arthur Sackler also helped himself in the process. For years, he had watched his pharmaceutical advertising clients grow rich. Their products often cost pennies to manufacture but were sold at huge markups. Sackler wanted a piece of the business but he faced a dilemma. He couldn't go into competition with his advertising clients, so he did the next best thing: he financed the purchase of a drug company and let his brothers run it.

In 1952 the Sacklers acquired a firm that was barely more than a shell company, with annual revenues of only $22,000. Located on Christopher Street in New York's Greenwich Village, it was called the Purdue Frederick Company.

The roots of Purdue Frederick stretch back to 1892, a time when entrepreneurs by the hundreds produced feel-good elixirs and patent medicines that owed their revitalizing or curative powers to opiates, alcohol, or some combination of the two. Founded by Dr. John Purdue Gray and George Frederick Bingham, one of the company's biggest sellers over the next several decades was a cure-all called Gray's Glycerine Tonic Compound, which contained a generous serving of sherry. A Purdue Frederick advertising card sent to physicians in 1937 read:

Dear Doctor

When Spring Comes Gray's Glycerine Tonic Comp. should be a suggestion to your patient—tired from Winter Ills. Prescribe this dependable Tonic which has stood "The Test of Time" for over forty-five (45) years.

Purdue's first products under Sackler-family management hardly suggested that one day it would produce powerful painkillers like OxyContin. In 1955, Purdue started selling a brand of laxatives under the name Senokot and three years later added the prescription earwax remover Cerumenex to its product line. Both were successful and, years later, still were sold by the company.

It is likely that Arthur Sackler played a major role in acquiring those products for Purdue. He knew, based on his experience in the pharmaceutical industry, that as a small, privately held operation, the company would prosper only if it found opportunities or created niches unclaimed by big manufacturers. That way of thinking decades later apparently led his brothers to see opportunity in one such overlooked area—the treatment of pain.

Back in the 1950s, however, Purdue Frederick was but one of several drug-related businesses that Mortimer and Raymond Sackler ran, and laxatives and earwax remover were but two products among their medical merchandise. They also owned the Glutavite Corporation, which sold a product called l-Glutavite. Advertisements for it that appeared in the *Medical*

Tribune depicted aging men and women and described l-Glutavite as a "metabolic cerebral tonic" capable of revitalizing
confused minds. Despite its quasi-medical name and claims of
restorative powers, l-Glutavite was a throwback to the era
of patent medicines. It was nothing more than a mixture
of monosodium glutamate—the meat tenderizer known as
MSG—and vitamin B. Not surprisingly, the ads promoting it
as a mental stimulant were the handicraft of the burgeoning
drug industry's dream factory, the William Douglas McAdams
agency, Arthur Sackler's firm.

By the late 1950s, ads like those for l-Glutavite and the ex-
plosive growth of the drug marketing industry had caught the
attention of an investigative journalist named John Lear. He believed that the promotional onslaught was corrupting the judg-
ments of doctors and posing threats to the public's health. In
the 1950s, for instance, antibiotics producers heavily promoted
the use of differing antibiotics at the same time to treat a patient, a dangerous practice that can create drug-resistant bac-
teria. Lear, then the science editor of the influential weekly
magazine *Saturday Review*, was horrified by what he saw and
began a series of investigative articles over the course of several
years that sought to unravel the increasingly intertwining
worlds of drug production and promotion.

Decades earlier, Lear had made his reputation by exposing
a major scandal in which an Agriculture Department official
had participated in a scheme that had bilked $2.6 million from
a government program meant to compensate farmers who were
forced to slaughter tubercular cattle. Lear showed that pay-

ments were made for cattle that didn't exist. Now, the reporting trail he was following led him straight toward the drug industry behemoth controlled by Arthur, Mortimer, and Raymond Sackler. John Lear quickly sensed their power within the drug industry. But he also soon suspected that it might extend into the very agency entrusted with regulating the drug industry, the FDA.

The linchpin in Lear's investigation was an FDA official named Henry Welch. Lear discovered that Welch, who was in charge of the agency's division that regulated antibiotics, was on the payroll of two journals that published research reports about such drugs, *Antibiotics and Chemotherapy* and *Antibiotic Medicine and Clinical Therapy*. Welch insisted when challenged by Lear that his ties to the publications did not pose a conflict of interest because the journals were independent. But a congressional investigation prompted by a Lear article in a 1959 issue of the *Saturday Review* found that the FDA official had in fact received some $287,000 in income over a six-year period through the publications, income that came from the very antibiotic producers whom Welch regulated. Those manufacturers had spent millions buying reprinted articles from the publications, which they then distributed as sales tools to doctors. The funds received by Welch reflected his cut of the take, a 7½ percent royalty. Not incidentally, drugmakers got to read and edit research articles about their antibiotics before they appeared in print.

Welch immediately resigned in disgrace. But Lear continued digging and discovered that the drug company payments for reprints from *Antibiotics and Chemotherapy* and *Antibiotic Medicine and Clinical Therapy* had been made to a company called MD Publications, which then paid Welch his share. The president of MD Publications was a researcher named Dr. Felix Marti-Ibanez, but Lear suspected that Marti-Ibanez was just a figurehead used to shield the true owners. For one, he was an employee of a branch of Sackler's advertising agency, and MD Publications shared office space with that firm. Marti-Ibanez had also worked with the Sackler brothers at Creedmoor. In addition, according to Lear's article, Henry Welch had said that Marti-Ibanez shared ownership of MD Publications with two investors whose identities he did not know. John Lear thought he had a pretty good idea of who they might be.

In a March 1962 issue he introduced readers of the *Saturday Review* to the Sackler brothers. He depicted them as modern-day moguls who had laid claim to the new industry of drug promotion with a tenacity akin to John D. Rockefeller's dominance of the oil industry or Jay Gould's seizure of the railroads. No doubt, Arthur, Mortimer, and Raymond took strong exception to the characterization, but exactly how they felt was anybody's guess; Lear's article gives no indication that they spoke with him.

Lear started the article by describing the Sackler brothers' production, promotion, and advertising of l-Glutavite as emblematic of the far greater transformation taking place throughout the pharmaceutical industry—its evolution into a mass-marketing machine for pills. Of them, he wrote:

The spectacle of three psychiatrists, members of a profession looked to with almost awesome respect for guidance in mental illness, concertedly pushing a flavoring extract mixed with vitamins as a means of arresting the pitiable deterioration of aging minds, is a painful experience. But the l-Glutavite episode has significance beyond the compass of psychiatry. It illustrates the machine-like disregard of individuality in which the once precise art of prescription drug administration has descended in America.

The combined resources of the three Sackler brothers for this type of integrated drug marketing were not exhausted in the promotion of l-Glutavite. The brothers cover every aspect of prescription medicine. They have succeeded in carrying out their operation despite opposition within the medical profession. Whatever opposition they may have encountered within the drug industry itself has not been effective.

Lear then set out in the article to make his case for a link between Henry Welch, MD Publications, and the Sacklers. He tried to piece together a tangled business trail, one all the more impenetrable because the companies involved were private and so didn't have to disclose their true ownership. But names involved with the Sacklers kept popping up, including that of a lawyer and an accountant who had done work for Arthur. Lear also noted that a news agency owned by Arthur was the first to announce in 1951 that Welch would edit a new journal called *Antibiotics and Chemistry*. In addition, Lear reported that Mortimer Sackler had sat on the editorial board of another antibiotics-related publication whose research articles had been cited in the ad created by William Douglas McAdams for the antibiotic Sigmamycin, the very ad that featured the business cards for doctors who didn't exist. Welch had cited Sigmamycin when, as an FDA official, he had announced the dawn of a new era of increased antibiotics use; several years later, the FDA sent a warning out to doctors that the drug was causing jaundice and liver damage.

But Lear could never find the proverbial smoking gun that directly tied any of the Sacklers to MD Publications. The thicket of corporate paperwork and tangled business dealings surrounding MD Publications was just too dense to penetrate. If Lear had proved his case, the carefully constructed world of Arthur Sackler might have tumbled down in 1962; as it was, he and his brothers soon left John Lear behind.

After its takeover by the Sacklers in 1952, Purdue Frederick became a small but very profitable business and Mortimer and Raymond Sackler, through a variety of business enterprises, became extremely wealthy. The drug company hit a home run when in 1966 it acquired a line of antiseptic products sold under the brand name Betadine, best known to consumers as the orange-colored disinfectant used widely by hospitals to scrub down patients prior to surgery. For Purdue, it was an ideal product, one with low production costs and high profit margins. In 1969, Betadine even enjoyed a fleeting moment of fame when astronaut Neil Armstrong used the solution to decontaminate the Apollo landing module after his historic moon walk.

By the 1970s the Sacklers' business operations had expanded overseas, and Mortimer and Raymond Sackler were living on different sides of the Atlantic. Raymond, who remained in Connecticut, became most closely associated with Purdue Frederick, the company's American arm. Mortimer was principally responsible for the family's European operations, including a British company called Napp Pharmaceuticals, which essentially was Purdue's English counterpart. Over time, the Sacklers would develop ties to pharmaceutical companies worldwide, including ones operating in such countries as Australia, Canada, Germany, and Japan.

But it was Napp's acquisition of a Scottish drug producer, Bard Laboratories, that set the stage for the company's move into pain treatment. Bard researchers had developed a sustained-release technology suitable for morphine, and Napp in 1980 began selling that drug in England under the brand name MST. Four years later, after the completion of the more rigorous testing required of new drugs by the FDA, the same drug was released by Purdue Frederick in the United States as MS Contin, the morphine-based predecessor to OxyContin.

By that time, Mortimer and Raymond Sackler were sixty-eight and sixty-four years old, respectively. They would continue to remain lifelong business partners, though by all accounts the two men had vastly different personalities and lifestyles. According to one mutual acquaintance, they also clashed at times; for instance, during Purdue board meetings they sat separated from each other by their lawyers. Acquaintances frequently described Raymond as quiet and retiring, and his first marriage endured. Mortimer was outgoing and loved the swirl of high society. He, like his older brother, Arthur, married three times, twice to far-younger women.

But unlike Arthur, who was known even to his friends as a tightwad, Mortimer lived large and enjoyed his many luxuries. In time, he owned palatial homes in London, the English countryside, the French Riviera town of Cap d'Antibes, and an Austrian resort village in the Alps. During summer days on the Riviera, guests regularly arrived in the late afternoon to join Mortimer in backgammon games played on the villa's rear patio. A tennis coach was on staff to give lessons to the Sacklers and their guests. In the winter the action moved to the Alps, where Mortimer hired skiing instructors. He lavished expensive gifts on his wives. In his second wife's vast collection of jewelry were two sets of Bulgari earrings valued at $480,000.

Mortimer's generosity extended beyond his wives and guests; with his brother Raymond he was a major donor to British art museums, including the British Museum, the Ashmolean Museum, the Serpentine Gallery, and other scientific and medical institutions. Along with the Metropolitan Museum, Raymond and Mortimer Sackler donated generously to various institutions in this country, including the Guggenheim Museum.

But Mortimer Sackler's decision to live in Europe may have been due to more than just business and an appreciation of the good life. His second wife, Gertraud, or "Geri," as she was known, was Austrian by birth, and in court papers she filed in 1984 following a bitter divorce battle between them, she explained her husband's decision to leave the United States this way:

> Mortimer D. Sackler, who was born in Brooklyn, New York, renounced his American citizenship in year 1974 and became a citizen of Austria and a resident of various countries in Europe. This was admittedly done by him to avoid paying United States taxes on his income in the United States as well as abroad.

One close intimate of Arthur Sackler said that he became furious when he learned that his brother had given up citizenship. "He kept saying, 'This is a great country. You started your business in this country,'" that person later recalled. Years later, Geri Sackler offered another reason for her former husband's decision—he felt a strong emotional tie to Austria because his parents had lived in eastern Europe before their immigration to the United States.

As for Mortimer Sackler, his court papers were silent about his U.S. citizenship and, years later, in responding to a list of questions about his citizenship, one of his lawyers replied, "Dr. Sackler will not respond to the questions you ask, except to advise you that the assumptions that underlie your questions are incorrect."

Whatever the case, by the time OxyContin went to market in the mid-1990s, Mortimer had long been married to his third wife and spent most of the year living in London. He traveled to the United States only occasionally to attend Purdue board meetings or art world events.

The memorial tribute for Arthur Sackler in 1987 was held at the Temple of Dendur at the Metropolitan Museum of Art. "He was a truly good person, a fine, splendid, noble human being with absolute integrity," his third wife, Gillian, said at the service. "He never had a small, devious, or petty thought."

During his later years, Sackler had sought to conquer the art world with the same determination and brushes with controversy that marked his business career. While making major donations to the Metropolitan Museum of Art, for instance, he used a museum storage room as a personal warehouse for his ever-growing collection of antiquities. But while a formidable collector, Arthur Sackler's quest for recognition as a cultural mandarin was never successful; some saw too little joy in his acquisitive nature. "He had the charm of the dollar sign," one auction house executive told *Vanity Fair* magazine shortly after Sackler's death.

Sackler had spent his life keeping many of his and his brothers' business dealings well hidden, and he expected, no doubt, that those secrets would follow him into the grave. But

Arthur Sackler's death set off a brutal, nearly decade-long legal battle between Gillian, who was known as "Jill," and his four children over his vast estate. She wasn't their mother but a woman not that much older than themselves whom their father had met while she was working as a secretary in the London offices of the *Medical Tribune*.

The amount of money involved was massive; while Sackler's estate was valued in legal papers at $140 million, one of his former financial advisers estimated its worth at many times that amount. And while his heirs fought over those spoils, nearly fifteen bankers' boxes of legal documents would begin to fill the shelves in a Long Island courthouse.

Some of the Sackler brothers' best-kept secrets about business ventures, including Purdue, spilled out in court papers. For example, Arthur Sackler had long portrayed himself as a fierce competitor of Ludwig Wilhelm Frohlich, who ran L. W. Frohlich Inc., the other dominant drug-advertising agency of the 1950s and 1960s. However, court papers showed that he, his two brothers, and Frohlich were apparently collaborators and partners. Indeed, in a memo Sackler wrote in 1973, he referred to "properties jointly built between myself, Mr. Frohlich and my brothers."

Among those ventures was IMS, the prescription tracking company that Purdue would later use to identify doctors who were writing prescriptions for OxyContin. As far as the public knew, Frohlich was the owner and head of IMS. But the idea for IMS came from Arthur Sackler, or so Arthur's children and lawyer would claim. And as with much else in the brothers' world, Mortimer and Raymond were partners in the business.

At a meeting of the trustees of his estate, Michael Sonnenreich, Arthur Sackler's lawyer and longtime confidant, explained that "under the four-way agreement, [Arthur] gave away his rights to IMS. . . . But his understanding with Frohlich was that if he ever sold it, he was entitled to one-fourth."

That never happened, according to Arthur's daughter Elizabeth. And during that same trustees' meeting, she railed at her uncles for cutting her father out of the money due him from IMS when the company went public.

"Dad came up with the idea for IMS, and on a handshake with Bill Frohlich, Bill was given the go-ahead," she said, according to the minutes of that trustees' meeting. "I don't know a lot of the intermediary steps that happened, but I know that when Frohlich died, Raymond and Morty made out like bandits when the stock went public. As I understood it, Dad received nothing."

Jill Sackler also claimed that Raymond and Mortimer had helped themselves to profits from Purdue Frederick that should have gone to their older brother, according to estate records. "There was supposed to be a three-way agreement with Purdue Frederick, and they have taken gigantic sums out of that," she told Sonnenreich during another trustees' meeting.

It fell to Sonnenreich to untangle a lifetime of business dealings between Arthur Sackler and his brothers. In some cases, Mortimer and Raymond transferred business assets in which Arthur held an interest back into their brother's estate for the benefit of his heirs. In other cases, they purchased those holdings from the estate for themselves. Long before the battle between Arthur's children and Jill Sackler was settled, a deal was struck under which Mortimer and Raymond agreed to pay the estate $22,353,750 for their brother's one-third stake in Purdue.

John Lear, the science journalist who tried in the 1960s to penetrate the Sacklers' wall of silence, never had a chance to sort through those courthouse records. He died in 1999, apparently unaware that they even existed.

Had he known about them, Lear would have discovered that much of what he had suspected about Arthur Sackler and his brothers was right. For instance, these very estate papers contained the evidence he had been looking for: documents that indicated the Sacklers owned MD Publications, the company that funneled some $260,000 in reprint royalty payments to Henry Welch, the compromised FDA official. The ownership of the company may have bounced around; for example, court records indicated that Mortimer and Raymond or entities they controlled may have held stakes in it and, as Lear suspected, may have been the two mysterious unidentified stockholders. But the final resting place for MD Publications in Arthur's estate spoke loudly enough. As Win Gerson, the top executive at William Douglas McAdams, told a lawyer trying to understand Sackler's business dealings, "To me, the whole thing was Arthur."

By that time, Mortimer and Raymond Sackler were

preparing OxyContin for its launch. Forty years had passed since Mortimer and Raymond Sackler had started their pharmaceutical careers peddling l-Glutavite, the "metabolic cerebral tonic." During that time, they had amassed enormous wealth. They had given generously to museums and medical institutions. The Sackler name was now engraved on cultural and educational temples throughout the world. Adversaries like John Lear had been vanquished long ago.

But now in 2001, near the end of their lives, Mortimer and Raymond Sackler faced one last threat to their legacy. Arthur Sackler had been an original and a visionary; he'd been bold, brilliant, and larger than life. Mortimer's and Raymond's feelings toward him must have been complex, a mixture of gratitude and envy, love and resentment.

Now, with OxyContin, they were facing a challenge that would have tested even Arthur Sackler's extraordinary abilities. But this time Arthur wasn't around to help; Mortimer and Raymond, their children, and their retinue of advisers were on their own. They would have to remember and rely on every skill that Arthur Sackler had tried to teach them. Their success would serve as his ultimate bequest.

CHAPTER TEN

THE BODY COUNT

ON AN APRIL DAY IN 2002, there was an electric feeling inside the normally sober offices of the DEA. Laura Nagel was ready to drop a bombshell on Purdue. An agency pharmacologist had just handed her the ammunition she'd been looking for.

The scientist, Dave Gauvin, had been spending the last few months hunched inside his tiny office cubicle sifting through the 1,300 separate death reports sent into DEA following the agency's request the previous summer for data on oxycodone-related overdoses. Gauvin, a large, heavyset man, had discarded around 350 of the reports because they didn't contain enough information to be useful in the analysis he was conducting. The remaining 950 reports had been analyzed and put into a database that was intended to determine how often OxyContin had been the source of the oxycodone detected during autopsies and toxicological examinations.

Laura Nagel had always suspected it would be high, but what Gauvin told her exceeded her expectations. His analysis showed that OxyContin itself was either definitely or very likely to have been involved in one-half of all cases. To arrive at that figure, the DEA researcher had broken down the reported overdose fatalities into groups, classifying some 145 cases, or about 15 percent of those reviewed, as "OxyContin verified" because medical reports or police information showed that an OxyContin tablet or prescription had been found at the autopsy or at the death scene. He deemed another 318 deaths, or 34 percent of the cases analyzed, as "OxyContin-likely." That category constituted those cases in which toxicology tests run on overdose victims had detected oxycodone but not aspirin or acetaminophen, the nonprescription analgesics used in Percocet, Tylox, and other oxycodone-containing painkillers. Since OxyContin accounted for 80 percent of all painkiller prescriptions written for medications that contained only the narcotic, Gauvin and DEA staffers concluded that it was a safe bet that the oxycodone found in those cases had also likely come from OxyContin. Half of all the cases were left unclassified because DEA researchers couldn't determine whether or not OxyContin was involved.

These were sobering statistics. But for Nagel it was Gauvin's other finding that was likely to change the entire face of the debate over the painkiller. The DEA analyst's study indicated that it wasn't just drug abusers and recreational users who were succumbing in OxyContin-related overdoses; pain patients had been dying too.

Gauvin based his conclusion on the mixes of different prescription drugs found during a number of autopsies. It wasn't at all unusual for a drug overdose death to involve multiple substances; in fact, it was the rare drug-related death, often a suicide, where only a single drug was found. But Gauvin's attention had turned to particular combinations of medications that kept showing up in many autopsy reports. Along with oxycodone, overdose victims at the time of their death often had other painkillers, tranquilizers, and antidepressants in their systems, or "on board," as toxicologists like to say. Gauvin knew that many patients who had chronic pain were prescribed such combinations of medications, and he took the findings as evidence that pain sufferers had also become part of the body count. Agency officials felt so strongly about these findings that they planned to submit them to a scientific journal for publication. Before that, however, the DEA issued a news release in April 2002, summing up its death data review and its apparent implications for pain patients:

A "normal" patient receiving a standard OxyContin prescription regimen approved by the Food and Drug Administration may be a poly-drug user. One treatment strategy recommended for "chronic pain" patients is the co-administration of opioids with anti-depressants—

225

again, a treatment strategy, by its design, results in poly-drug usage. With these facts in mind it was not surprising to find that many of the OxyContin deaths were associated with poly-drug toxicologies. This does not minimize the significance of OxyContin in these deaths.

Laura Nagel was convinced that when she presented FDA officials with evidence that legitimate pain patients were also dying, they'd be forced to take action. But things didn't turn out that way. Instead, when Purdue executives and FDA officials arrived at her office on a day in mid-April to be briefed about the DEA review, Nagel's bombshell blew up in her face.

As Nagel laid out her case, officials of the drugmaker dismissed the data out of hand, saying that there was nothing in it to scientifically support her suggestion that pain patients were overdosing. Purdue scientists pointed out, for instance, that the mere discovery of OxyContin and a tranquilizer like Valium together at autopsy could just as easily mean that drug abusers took the medications together to customize their high. They also vehemently disputed that the DEA data showed that Oxy-Contin itself was causing fatal overdoses.

Dr. Cynthia McCormick, one of the FDA officials who played a leading role in negotiating changes to OxyContin's label, was also at the DEA meeting, and she sided with Purdue's stance. She believed that the death reports reviewed by the DEA were just too ambiguous to arrive at any conclusions about the safety of OxyContin; instead, it was the FDA's position that OxyContin was safe when taken as directed.

"We don't believe there is cause for panic," an FDA official told the *New York Times* after the meeting.

For Nagel, the experience was a crushing one. She had been caught out of her depth and there was nothing for her to fall back on. As a cop, she had viewed the death data in terms of black and white, but the picture offered by the medical examiners' reports was far murkier. It was a rookie's mistake, and a big one. The DEA had never attempted such an ambitious forensic analysis before. While some of Gauvin's statistical findings would prove to be accurate, he'd leapt to a conclusion about overdose deaths in pain patients that the data couldn't support.

Nagel's defeat would continue to sting. FDA officials would later say that the DEA never shared its autopsy data as it had originally promised. DEA officials said it was available but that their FDA counterparts never came to review it. Whatever the case, the episode was an embarrassment for Nagel that she didn't want and couldn't afford to repeat.

As she would later say, "It was the worst day of my life."

Laura Nagel wasn't the only one of Purdue's adversaries who stumbled in 2002. Indeed, with each passing month there was a palpable sense that the tide had turned in the drugmaker's favor.

In February, for instance, Art Van Zee and Sue Ella Kobak went to Washington so that Art could testify at a hearing about OxyContin held by the Senate Health, Education and Pensions

Committee, which was chaired by Massachusetts Senator Edward Kennedy. Van Zee had never appeared in front of federal lawmakers and it struck him that the hearing was perhaps his last and best shot to have an impact on the drug's use.

But as he and Sue Ella drove to the nation's capital in their 1999 Dodge van, she sensed that her husband was growing more nervous by the mile.

"What are the most important points I can make?" he kept asking her. "I only have five minutes. What are the three most important points I should make?"

They stopped over the first night in Richmond, Virginia, where they hooked up with Sam Church, a family friend who was a top lobbyist for the United Mine Workers of America. Patti Church, Sam's wife, worked for Sue Ella as a legal secretary, and her husband had arranged for Van Zee to testify through his contacts with Senator John Warner of Virginia.

The following day, when Van Zee arrived at a Senate hearing room, he was wearing his only suit, a blue one. He had on a colorful Jerry Garcia necktie that his mother had given to him. Both Church and Sue Ella were there to lend Art support, but the physician was so nervous that he kept disappearing every few minutes to go to the bathroom. Several Purdue executives also entered the hearing, including Dr. Paul Goldenheim, a top company scientist who was set to testify. The company contingent cordially greeted Van Zee and took their seats.

When his turn came to speak, the Lee County physician repeated his argument that Purdue should be required to recall its drug until it could be reformulated.

"My own personal view of the complicated OxyContin abuse problem is that there are at least three major elements involved," he told the Senate panel. "First, there has been an obvious problem with physician misprescribing and overprescribing of this drug. Secondly, this epidemic has been a vicious indicator of the alarming degree of prescription drug abuse in this society. Thirdly, and perhaps the one closest to this committee and the FDA, is that the promotion and marketing of OxyContin by Purdue Pharma has played a major role in this problem."

In their questions and comments, members of the Senate panel made it clear that they didn't intend to take specific actions against the painkiller. But Senator Christopher Dodd of Connecticut, the home state of Purdue, kept challenging Van Zee to provide evidence showing that the drugmaker's promotion of OxyContin had spurred its abuse. Dodd pointed out to Van Zee that it seemed to him that the crisis in places like Lee County involved a long-standing problem with prescription drugs that extended well beyond OxyContin.

"There is something far more profound going on here than just the availability through legal channels of a painkiller," Dodd commented.

Van Zee responded that he didn't have all the information to prove his point. But he added that he believed that when a drug company aggressively promoted narcotics to doctors who were already high prescribers of such substances in areas known for prescription drug abuse, it was a "recipe for commercial success and public health problems."

In a written statement accompanying his testimony, Dr. Goldenheim described a litany of steps the company had taken to respond to the OxyContin episode, including changes to the product's label, drug abuse prevention programs aimed at children, and Purdue's increased efforts to work jointly with medical and law enforcement groups.

Dr. Goldenheim, a thin man with graying hair and a mustache, also disputed the notion that Purdue had promoted its drug too aggressively. Some months earlier, several public officials had attacked the company for doing so, pointing to, among other things, a pen that Purdue distributed to doctors containing a pull-down chart that showed the strengths the doctors should use when converting patients on other pain medications to OxyContin.

The officials had charged that the pen showed Purdue was pushing doctors to use OxyContin in place of other pain medications less prone to abuse. But Dr. Goldenheim, in his testimony, refuted that.

"The notion that these conversion charts are an attempt to encourage physicians to switch patients to OxyContin from less abusable drugs is unfounded," Goldenheim said in his statement. "These charts are intended, and understood, by physicians, to be used when those lower scheduled [less abuse prone] drugs are not working."

Purdue marketing documents that were publicly disclosed about a year later showing that the drugmaker aimed to convince doctors to use OxyContin even before trying other, lower-scheduled narcotics, or even Ultram, a non-narcotic. But whatever the case, it was clear by the hearing's end that Art Van Zee hadn't swayed anyone.

In closing the session, Rhode Island Senator Jack Reed thanked Van Zee, Paul Goldenheim, and the other witnesses for helping the panel to better understand the complex issues surrounding pain treatment and narcotics abuse. "I suspect we'll continue to think about and worry about these issues going forward," Reed said.

Late that afternoon, Art and Sue Ella piled back in their van for the long drive back to Lee County. Van Zee's quixotic quest appeared to have run out of steam; no lawmakers seemed to be interested in taking up the issue of OxyContin. Still, Sue Ella had a few souvenirs of the trip. While she and Sam Church waited for the hearing to start, they had wandered into a conference room where she noticed a pile of disposable coasters emblazoned with the seal of the United States Senate. She told Church she liked them, but when she looked for the coasters again they had disappeared. She figured that Sam Church had pocketed them, and when Sue Ella asked him about it he turned the loot over to her. Back in Lee County, Sue Ella gave one of the coasters to an uncle who lived in a nursing home, telling him that Senator Warner had sent it to him. Sue Ella's uncle was so proud of the coaster that years later he'd still be using it.

Purdue's victories in 2002 came not only on the political front but in the courtroom as well. The drugmaker began to easily swat aside some of the personal injury lawsuits brought against it, such as the Kentucky case in which Art Van Zee had testified.

The contests were largely mismatches. The burst of newspaper articles about OxyContin's abuse and its addictive potential had set off a courthouse stampede led by small-town and small-time plaintiffs' lawyers who sensed an easy opportunity. But they soon found themselves facing two of the biggest corporate defense law firms in the United States, King & Spalding of Atlanta and Chadbourne & Parke of New York City. Purdue had hired the firms to manage its legal defense, and their depth of resources and legal talent was formidable; both had also defended cigarette makers in cases brought against them.

Along with facing formidable adversaries, some plaintiffs' lawyers suing Purdue confronted another problem—their own clients. Some were people who had abused other drugs before OxyContin and so were hardly likely to win the sympathies of jurors. As a result, plaintiffs' lawyers were forced to scramble to find new clients whom they hoped to show had innocently wandered into the world of abuse and addiction through the gateway of OxyContin.

With each lawsuit dismissal in 2002, Purdue officials issued a celebratory news release, laden with saber rattling.

"These dismissals strengthen our resolve to defend these cases vigorously and to the hilt," general counsel Howard Udell said in one August announcement. "We have not settled one of these cases—not one. Personal injury lawyers who bring them in the hopes of a quick payday will continue to be disappointed."

Such victories, however, weren't coming cheap. In September, Udell told a legal publication, *Corporate Counsel*, that the company had already spent $45 million on legal expenses and its legal bills were mounting at the monthly rate of about $3 million. Meanwhile, the company was still swamped by lawsuits; even with a series of rapid dismissals, more than a hundred OxyContin-related claims against the company remained.

Meanwhile, Purdue's multimillion-dollar effort to reshape public opinion about the company and its drug was forging ahead. That initiative had started in areas hardest hit by OxyContin's abuse even before the onslaught of news about the painkiller in the early spring of 2001. Ever since then, the drugmaker had been spending lavishly and recruiting aggressively in an effort to forge links with individuals or organizations outside its traditional base in the pain management community.

Back in March 2001, for instance, an internal memo shows that the drugmaker was scheduled to hold talks with Dr. Lewis W. Sullivan, the former head of the federal Department of Health and Human Services, about the possibility of hiring him as the company's national pain management spokesperson. While that arrangement never materialized, the company did soon retain Dr. Sullivan to advise Purdue on the development of medical school courses on pain treatment and drug abuse monitoring.

Jay McCloskey, one of the company's original critics, also soon signed on as a consultant on legal and drug abuse prevention issues. McCloskey began working for Purdue in May

2001, soon after he left his prosecutor's post. But the same memo that cited the drugmaker's contact with Dr. Sullivan indicates that McCloskey may have contacted Purdue about future work two months earlier, a time when he was still in public office. The memo, which was dated March 21, 2001, and entitled "Actions Underway," was a rundown of efforts undertaken at the time by Purdue in various states and at the federal level, including scheduled meetings with public officials. With respect to Maine, the document states:

> a) AG [Maine's state attorney general] wants to take over our relationship [as the point person on the OxyContin issue] now that McCloskey is leaving. RH to call and schedule a meeting.
> b) We will try to schedule a follow-up with McCloskey while we are there; he called looking for business for his new law practice.
> c) News release put out on 3/8 on tamper-resistant prescription pad program; McCloskey prepped to field questions and compliment PPLP [Purdue Pharma] for our initiative in "doing the right thing."

Years later, McCloskey vehemently disputed any suggestion that he had contacted the company seeking work prior to leaving his prosecutor's job. Whatever the case, Jay McCloskey was hardly the only former public official who would eventually find him- or herself on Purdue's payroll, either as an employee or a consultant. The company hired a number of local law enforcement officials from states like Virginia and also retained former DEA agents. Purdue also began increasing its ties to and involvement with professional organizations such as the National Association of Drug Diversion Investigators. The group represented local and federal drug agents, including many who had dealt firsthand with OxyContin's abuse.

At the group's annual meeting in 2001, for example, David Haddox presented investigators with a slide show picturing newspaper reports that the Purdue physician said had overstated either the scope of the OxyContin problem or the drug's addictive potential. Some law enforcement officials saw Haddox's presentation as an effort at damage control. One DEA diversion investigator who attended Haddox's talk recalled how a prosecutor from Tennessee passed a note during it that read, "This is like Philip Morris saying that cigarettes don't cause cancer."

Increasingly, however, Haddox and other Purdue executives and consultants became fixtures at meetings of the National Association and the company's contributions to the organization grew. Officers of the group said that they believed the drug-maker's role was a positive one and that company officials never tried to set the organization's agenda. But Laura Nagel, among others, didn't like what she was hearing. Her solution: in 2002 she sharply reduced the number of DEA agents allowed to attend the organization's meetings.

Purdue's efforts to influence public officials didn't stop with the law enforcement group. At its annual convention in 2002, the National Association of State Controlled Substances Authorities, a group of state-level drug regulators, was entertained by Eric B. Dezenhall, a principal of the corporate crisis management firm hired by Purdue to "manage" the OxyContin crisis. The title of his talk: "Who Survives the Media and Why."

Dezenhall's presentation was a marked change of pace from the message that the same group had heard just two years ago from one of its own. Its theme: a prescription narcotics disaster was about to wreak havoc in the lives of both young people and pain patients.

At a gathering of the National Association of State Controlled Substances Authorities in 2000, John Eadie, a New York State official, warned his colleagues as well as drug industry executives like David Haddox that urgent action was needed to avert a calamity. Eadie told the group that federal survey data showed that young people were now experimenting with legal narcotics in numbers so alarming that they paralleled the worst years of the cocaine epidemic of the 1980s.

A failure to act, Eadie warned, would lead to the creation of a new generation of lifetime drug abusers as well as a social backlash toward the use of narcotics that would imperil the legitimate medical needs of pain patients.

Eadie wrote in the group's newsletter that if the problem "is not reversed quickly" then there was a high risk of injuring "a very significant number of children and young adults through accidents, addiction, overdoses and death."

Two years later, John Eadie's unheeded warning would be forgotten amidst the rush to make over Purdue's corporate image.

And in 2002, the drugmaker added a true star to the ranks of those enlisted to aid that effort. Robin Hogen, its top spokesman, could barely contain himself as he described to fellow public relations executives the forthcoming announcement and the change in Purdue's corporate strategy toward dealing with the OxyContin controversy that it represented.

"I have to admit that our company looked like food for about the first year of this crisis," Hogen said in March 2002. "We were quite reactive, we were kind of stunned. We were saying, well, look at the science, look at the data, read the literature. And we were trying to argue with scientific arguments in what became a political war. And we had to switch over to using more political consultants in fact. And we're about to announce next week bringing on a sort of rock star in that area. I can't tell you today who it is, but we're going to be bringing on a very impressive individual who is a political star. That's all that I can tell you—because it's a political issue. And we'd like to think that there's a level playing field out there somewhere, and that science and truth will win the day. That, unfortunately, is not the truth, and, in fact, you have to be politically Machiavellian often to win the day. So that's the direction we are heading in."

Purdue soon unveiled the name of its political "rock star," and as far as former politicians go, they don't get much bigger. It was Rudolph W. Giuliani, the former mayor of New York City. Prior to September 11, Giuliani had himself been saddled with a Machiavellian political reputation. But as he guided a battered city back onto its feet in the days and months following that harrowing event, he had displayed a remarkable grit and determination that had won praise from even his staunchest critics.

In the process, Giuliani had transformed himself not only into a media star but also into a rising force within the Republican Party whose name by 2002 was being bandied about for higher office. But as he weighed his political future, he had decided to cash in on his newfound stature by opening a consulting firm called Giuliani Partners.

Drawing on his years as a federal prosecutor, Giuliani set himself up as a corporate "Mr. Clean" for hire, and troubled companies soon started flocking to his door. Along with Purdue, his other clients would grow to include WorldCom, the telecom giant that was mired in an accounting scandal; the National Thoroughbred Racing Association, which was enmeshed in a bid-rigging controversy; and Merrill Lynch, one of many Wall Street brokerage firms accused of misleading investors. The firm didn't disclose the fees it received, but Giuliani's name and advice didn't come cheap; on the lecture circuit, he commanded $100,000 for an after-dinner talk.

In announcing his hiring, Purdue executives said that they had enlisted Giuliani's firm to help them improve, among other things, security at the company's OxyContin manufacturing plant in Totowa, New Jersey, which was still the subject of a DEA investigation. And within Giuliani Partners, overall responsibility for that job fell to ex–New York City police commissioner Bernard B. Kerik, who had followed his boss into the private sector.

Giuliani, who had only recently recovered from prostate

cancer, issued a public statement supporting Purdue and its mission of managing pain.

"There are tens of millions of Americans suffering from persistent pain," Giuliani said in a prepared statement at the time of his hiring. "We must find a way to ensure access to appropriate prescription pain medications for those suffering from the debilitating effects of pain while working to prevent the abuse and diversion of these same vital medicines."

But as Robin Hogen had told fellow public relations executives on the eve of Giuliani's hiring, his biggest attraction to Purdue were his political skills. And soon both he and Bernard Kerik were in direct contact with Asa Hutchinson, the administrator of DEA and Laura Nagel's boss.

"The mayor and I just met with Asa Hutchinson, the director of the DEA, his staff, and people from Purdue," Bernard Kerik told *New York* magazine in 2002. "We don't want Purdue put in a position where it winds up being taken over by the courts. Or they get put out of business. What I'd like to see come out of this is we set model security standards for the industry." In the same article, the magazine noted that just a week prior to Kerik's comment, Giuliani had raised $15,000 in donations for a traveling museum operated by the DEA.

The growing discussions between Giuliani and Hutchinson created consternation among some DEA officials. Normally, the DEA's administrator rarely gets involved in manufacturing plant investigation; it is even rare for the head of the diversion office, the position that Laura Nagel held, to become deeply involved with such matters on an ongoing basis. Instead, the heads of the

DEA's local field officials refer cases they believe merit legal or administrative actions directly to the Justice Department, which makes the ultimate decision about how to proceed.

But with Giuliani now in the mix, the pace of DEA's investigation into Purdue's OxyContin plant in New Jersey slowed as Hutchinson repeatedly summoned division officials to his office to explain themselves and their reasons for continuing the inquiry. In the end, however, the investigation proceeded. By late 2002, Asa Hutchinson had left DEA to take a top post at the Department of Homeland Security. And after that, DEA officials rarely heard from Rudolph Giuliani and Bernard Kerik again.

Right around the time of Hutchinson's departure, Purdue executives would successfully resolve an even more pressing matter. A year earlier, Florida's attorney general, Bob Butterworth, had opened an inquiry that he said had two objectives: one, to determine whether Purdue had improperly promoted OxyContin; and two, to pinpoint just when officials of the drugmaker had first learned about the drug's abuse. At the time, Butterworth had said that he was launching his probe because of the large number of OxyContin-related deaths in his state.

"I got involved primarily because I was reading the reports of the deaths from the medical examiners," Butterworth told the *South Florida Sun-Sentinel*. "That sort of gets your attention."

Butterworth could be a formidable foe; just a few years earlier he was one of the attorneys general who had spearheaded the assault against the tobacco industry. The attorney general of West Virginia, Darrell McGraw Jr., had already filed a similar claim against Purdue, and Butterworth's investigation now loomed as the possible prelude to similar claims by public officials not only in Florida but elsewhere.

As it turned out, however, Butterworth's inquiry was hardly a model of investigative zeal. While his office obtained a list from Purdue that contained the names of some one hundred former and present sales reps, an investigator formally interviewed only one of them. In that interview, William Gergely, who had served as the company's district sales manager for eastern Pennsylvania and West Virginia, said that two Purdue marketing executives, Jim Lang and Russell Gasdia, had described OxyContin during a meeting with sales reps as "non-habit forming." Gergely, who was fired from Purdue in 2000 after a colleague filed a sexual harassment claim against him, also said that the weekend-long pain management seminars sponsored by the drugmaker were simply "junkets" that were used to recruit doctors as paid speakers so they could help boost OxyContin sales.

Despite such claims, the investigation stalled in the summer of 2002. After serving four terms as attorney general, Butterworth was blocked by state term limit laws from running again. As a result, he was poised to move on and soon announced a campaign bid for a seat in the Florida State Senate.

With Butterworth's departure from office and an election looming, there was increased pressure to resolve open investigations both to gain any political benefit and to eliminate the risk that a new attorney general would shut down the inquiry. And it was just four days before Floridians went to the polls that year that Butterworth and Purdue struck a deal. Under it, Purdue agreed to pay $2 million to Florida to help underwrite a prescription monitoring plan for use in the state, which did not have one. In exchange, Butterworth agreed to close his inquiry. Both sides applauded the deal.

"Today's agreement marks several historic firsts in our nation's battle to curb the illegal use and abuse of prescription drugs," Butterworth said at a press conference. He added that such medications can "improve life for millions of pain-suffering Americans, or end life for a growing number of Americans who use and abuse them illegally."

On Purdue's behalf, Howard Udell said he believed that a prescription monitoring system in Florida would benefit pain patients by making it harder for drug abusers to get narcotics through legal channels.

"It is becoming increasingly difficult for legitimate pain patients to get prescriptions," Udell told the *South Florida Sun-Sentinel*. "Today, we're doing something about that."

With the investigation ended, Butterworth and other state officials would characterize their new relationship with Purdue executives as one of partners rather than adversaries. Later, however, two interesting letters written just a few months before, while the investigation was still continuing, emerged. One of them was from an assistant Florida attorney general, Jody E. Collins, who had recently taken over the Purdue inquiry. The other letter was from a lawyer in Florida hired by Purdue.

In her August letter, Collins demanded that the company turn over to her documents bearing directly on the heart of the state's inquiry. For example, she wanted Purdue to furnish all records documenting precisely when Purdue executives and sales reps learned about OxyContin's abuse in Maine and Virginia, the states where it appeared the drug's problems had first surfaced. And Collins also wanted to know what Purdue officials had told each other about those problems.

Among other things, Collins told Purdue she wanted

> True copies of all communications, including but not limited to e-mails, memos, faxes, alerts and correspondence, regarding the increase in sales, usage and/or abuse of OxyContin in the states of Maine and Virginia, from the OxyContin launch date until January 31, 2000, a) between Purdue Pharma and those representatives, area managers, district managers, and supervisors responsible for the sales territories of Maine and Virginia, and b) between and among any other personnel, officers, directors or managers of Purdue Pharma.

But Collins never got that information or those answers. Instead, she received a letter from Jon A. Sale, a Florida lawyer who represented Purdue. It confirmed that Collins' inquiry had been put on hold because talks had started between Butterworth's office and Purdue that would eventually result in a settlement. Sale's letter read:

This is to acknowledge receipt of your document request dated August 19, 2002. This letter confirms our agreement permitting Purdue Pharma to abate and stay production of the documents requested in your letter during the pendency of settlement discussions.

As it turned out, 2002 was a very good year for Purdue. The company had spent tens of millions of dollars on the corporate world's best lawyers, crisis management consultants, public relations spin artists, and advertising to improve its corporate image. Its financial reach had extended beyond pain advocacy and medical groups into law enforcement organizations, and its employee ranks were increasingly being filled by former police officials and retired DEA agents. Rudolph Giuliani, a true political heavyweight, had joined the company's team, and Purdue executives had also turned to another time-honored political staple, campaign finance. The drugmaker formed a political action committee whose coffers were filled with contributions from Sackler family members, along with company executives and their spouses. The biggest individual recipient of political funds that year was Connecticut Senator Christopher Dodd, the lawmaker who had closely questioned Art Van Zee. Not long afterward, Dodd received $10,000 from Purdue, ten times the amount given to any other federal official that year. Communities hard hit by OxyContin also received financial grants from Purdue; for example, the funds spurned by the Lee Coalition were later accepted by an organization located not far from Pennington Gap.

Tens of millions might seem like a lot to spend, but for Purdue with its billion-dollar drug it was small change; in 2002 the company was selling nearly $30 million worth of Oxy-Contin every week. By comparison, its counterattack had scored big successes. Congress had been quieted. Laura Nagel had been humbled. Art Van Zee's crusade had fallen off the tracks. Even Bob Butterworth shared the fate of those who had crossed swords with Purdue; he lost his bid for the Florida State Senate, buried by a landslide.

Meanwhile, 2002 had also been a bad year for Lindsay Myers. Not long after her urine screen had proved positive for cocaine, everything went haywire. She was still going to the methadone clinic but she soon plunged headlong back into abusing Oxys and her life of petty crime began again. For a time she used the gasoline credit card her father had given her to cover the cost of filling up her friends' cars. In return, they would give her cash, which she then spent on drugs.

One day that spring she went to the funeral for the father of a boy she knew. Not long afterward, she broke up with Ray and started going out with him. Several months later, she told her parents that she was pregnant; her new boyfriend was the father.

Larry Lavender had been counseling Lindsay for the past year and even with her now constant relapses she kept seeing him because she liked and trusted Lavender. But he had started to really worry about her. Lindsay didn't know whether to let her pregnancy go forward or have an abortion; on several occasions she made appointments at a nearby abortion clinic but then never showed up. As her fear about the baby and her sense of hopelessness increased, so did her drug use. Her appetite seemed so insatiable that only an overdose would stop it. When Lavender looked at Lindsay he began to get frightened; he saw himself two decades earlier standing gun in hand on a stretch of Baltimore waterfront. He began to worry that Lindsay might kill herself.

Jane and Johnny were also in a panic, and they came to see Lavender to try to decide what to do. Lavender suggested that given Lindsay's fragile state, it might be best to put her into a long-term residential treatment program until her pregnancy was over. The Myerses agreed to the plan, and Lavender found a facility in Chattanooga that took in pregnant women.

In the fall of 2002, Lindsay's parents drove her to Tennessee, but when the people running the clinic told Jane that they would keep Lindsay on methadone until the baby was born, Jane got scared and brought Lindsay back home. It is standard treatment procedure for pregnant women to remain on methadone to prevent the onset of stressful withdrawal prior to childbirth. But Jane worried, as many people might, about the birth of an addicted grandchild.

Lindsay's drug taking didn't stop, though, and that put her baby at even greater risk. One day, Jane stopped by to see Lindsay at her boyfriend's house, where she was now living. But when she arrived, the boy told her that Lindsay wasn't there. She was in a nearby jail, after being charged a few hours earlier with shoplifting vials of nasal spray from a Wal-Mart. The boy said that his parents had already left to bail her out.

But even spending a few hours of her pregnancy in an orange jumpsuit didn't deter Lindsay. Soon, valuable jewelry started disappearing from the Myerses' home, including a diamond-studded ring that belonged to Johnny and a gold rope necklace that belonged to Brandon, Lindsay's brother. Jane's mother soon called her; an emerald ring with diamonds was missing from her house.

Lavender got a tip that Lindsay was pawning jewelry at a local video store. He passed the information on to Jane, who went down to the store and started buying the pieces back. Jane and Johnny came down together to see Larry. They decided that they couldn't allow their daughter's behavior to continue; the danger was too great for her and the baby. Now, more than just one life was at stake.

CHAPTER
ELEVEN

PURPLE PEELERS

EVER SINCE THE OXY-Contin controversy began, Purdue executives had insisted in sworn testimony and in interviews that there had been a defining moment, a clear bright line when they had become aware of the painkiller's abuse. While the precise month varied depending on the Purdue official speaking, they concurred that they had learned about it at the same time and in the same way as drug regulators, law enforcement officials, and the public—in early 2000 when Jay McCloskey issued his alert to Maine doctors.

Michael Friedman had testified to that in August 2001 when he appeared before congressional investigators probing the case of Dr. Richard Paolino in Pennsylvania. So had Dr. Paul Goldenheim when he testified in December 2001 in front of a different congressional subcommittee. Invariably, the Purdue executives likened their discovery of the painkiller's problems not to a slow, troubled awakening but rather to a sudden arousal.

"In some 17 years of marketing MS-Contin Tablets, a controlled-release form of morphine—a powerful opioid analgesic related to oxycodone—Purdue was aware of no unusual experience of abuse or diversion," Goldenheim said in written testimony. "Purdue had no reason to expect otherwise with OxyContin. Neither Purdue, nor the FDA, nor the DEA, nor the medical community anticipated the extent of this problem. It was in February of 2000 that Purdue was first alerted to reports of abuse and diversion of OxyContin in rural parts of Maine according to the U.S. Attorney in Maine."

To be sure, no one can say precisely when the abuse of Oxy-Contin gathered momentum. But one thing was certain: The bright line in the sand drawn by Purdue around February 2000 wasn't that bright or clear-cut after all. In fact, if congressional officials had the interest or if Laura Nagel had the authority or if Bob Butterworth had the time they all might have discovered a critical part of the tragedy that became OxyContin abuse. It was simply this: There were growing warning signs prior to Jay McCloskey's alert that fateful February that OxyContin was being misused and that its timed-release formulation wasn't stopping it. In fact, throughout 1999, several episodes came to the attention of company executives or sales reps that pointed in the same direction: Purdue's billion-dollar painkiller was fast becoming a sought after street drug.

In early 1999, for example, a crisis erupted at Purdue's headquarters following a California doctor's arrest on murder charges in connection with an alleged pill mill that dispensed a huge volume of OxyContin. Not long afterward, a Purdue sales rep in Florida reported to his superiors that he had heard that OxyContin abuse was rampant in one part of that state. And right around the same time, Dr. Richard Norton, the physician near Pennington Gap whose patients Larry Lavender was assessing, told a Purdue sales rep there that his patients were getting high by crushing and chewing OxyContin tablets. Recreational users of traditional painkillers have long used that method to get a quicker jolt from those drugs and Norton told the sales rep that the same thing was happening to OxyContin.

Meanwhile, Jay McCloskey of Maine, as it turned out, wasn't the first public official to issue a warning about Oxy-Contin's abuse. Two similar alarms were sounded in 1999, and at least one of them came to the drug company's attention.

An editor at the *Weirton Daily Times*, a small newspaper in Weirton, West Virginia, recalled how that paper was visited in the spring of 1999 by a man and a woman who introduced themselves as Purdue sales reps. The pair asked to see back issues of the publication so that they could copy two articles that had appeared that April. In those pieces, the head of the local narcotics task force, William Beatty, issued a public warning that a new drug scourge was taking hold in and around Weirton, which is located in the northern tip of West Virginia that lies between Ohio and Pennsylvania.

"Too much heroin and too many Oxycontins [*sic*] are hitting the streets in the Upper Ohio Valley," Beatty wrote in one article. "People can die very easily from either one."

Years later, David Haddox remarked during a pain treatment conference that the company had received some information about OxyContin's abuse prior to Jay McCloskey's warning, reports that he characterized as "dribs and drabs."

But in 1998, just as the drugmaker was launching its massive promotional effort for OxyContin, a detailed report and an associated editorial appeared in a prestigious medical journal that foretold what lay ahead. In fact, the editorial's writer declared that the study's implications were so significant that they "should ring alarm bells." That study's bottom line: timed-release painkillers were potentially more attractive to drug abusers, not less so, because their narcotic payload was stronger and pure.

It was a report that touched on a critical cornerstone of Purdue's marketing drive to convince doctors to prescribe Oxy-Contin. Drug officials might have missed it, but it is unlikely because the report appeared in the *Journal of the Canadian Medical Association*, a publication in a country where Purdue had business operations. Published in July 1998, the report and the accompanying editorial challenged notions about the increased safety of timed-release narcotics.

Scientists from the University of British Columbia had uncovered the problem in 1998 when they decided to do research on prescription drug abuse in the real world—in their case, in a seedy section of downtown Vancouver. As part of their study they interviewed drug dealers about which prescription medicines they were peddling and the prices those drugs brought on the street.

Canadian researchers reported that MS Contin turned up frequently in the black market and that it commanded the highest street price of any prescription narcotic. Intravenous drug users simply scraped off the outer coating of an MS Contin tablet to circumvent the timed-release mechanism before crushing and dissolving the pill and then injecting it to get a heroin-like high. On the streets of Vancouver, the scientists found, MS Contin tablets were called "peelers" and were described by the color—a 10-milligram-strength tablet, for instance, was known as a "green peeler," and a 30-milligram-strength tablet was called a "purple peeler."

Meanwhile, the accompanying editorial appearing in the same Canadian publication noted that the Vancouver research appeared to contradict safety claims being made for timed-release narcotics such as those used by the FDA when it approved OxyContin's special label. The article was written by Dr. Brian Goldman, a drug abuse expert and emergency room physician in Toronto, who wrote that the researchers

> appear to be among the first to publish evidence on the street value of controlled-release opioid preparations (so-called "peelers"). It has been argued previously that controlled-release preparations might be less desirable as drugs of abuse than immediate-release pharmaceuticals. The relatively high street price of controlled-release opioid analgesics reported in this study clearly indicates that

these drugs are coveted. This should ring alarm bells. The manufacturer of one brand of morphine sulfate tablets (MS Contin) has warned that injection of the drug obtained by street crude methods could result in local tissue necrosis and pulmonary granuloma [conditions produced by the injection of talc, which is used as a binding agent in the manufacture of pharmaceutical tablets]. These issues need to be resolved. Now that controlled-release oxycodone [OxyContin] has been licensed in Canada, we can expect that it and other controlled-release opioid analgesics will also find their way onto the black market.

As it would turn out, few physicians in this country would ever see those reports.

In February 1999, about six months after the appearance of the Canadian study, police officials and state drug agents stormed the offices of a pain clinic in the rural northern California town of Redding. Dr. Frank Fisher, the clinic's operator, as well as the owners of a local drugstore that had filled hundreds of Oxy-Contin prescriptions for Fisher's patients, were arrested. They were all charged with murder in connection with the deaths of three of Fisher's patients from drug overdoses that involved oxycodone, as well as for conspiring to defraud California of $2 million by filing false medical claims.

The case against the Redding doctor spilled out during court hearings that spring and foreshadowed others involving physicians charged with illegally prescribing OxyContin that would soon follow. California state prosecutors charged that Fisher had run a pill mill where the painkiller was a drug of choice. Data showed, for example, that Fisher in 1998 wrote a startling 46 percent of all the prescriptions for 80-milligram-strength OxyContin tablets issued to low-income patients enrolled in a state program, Medi-Cal. And the drugstore used by many of his patients, the Shasta Pharmacy, had purchased nearly four times the volume of oxycodone-containing painkillers like OxyContin than any other retail drugstore in the country, according to DEA statistics.

As Gary Binkerd, the state prosecutor, said, "It is the staggering amounts of this drug that were made available and under circumstances where it was reasonably foreseeable that these drugs would leak on to and become part of the illicit street market that forms the basis of the homicide charge." The drugstore's owners denied any wrongdoing, while Fisher maintained that his narcotics prescribing practices reflected new medical views about the need to use such drugs more aggressively in pain treatment.

The turmoil created in early 1999 by the abrupt closure of Fisher's practice foreshadowed similar problems elsewhere. Following the shut down of a physician's practice, those using drugs like OxyContin appropriately or inappropriately would flood area hospital emergency rooms in the grip of intense withdrawal symptoms. And legitimate pain patients, finding themselves without care, were often forced to contact pain advocacy groups or troll the Internet to find the name of a physician to treat them.

The news of Fisher's arrest was widely reported in California newspapers such as the *San Francisco Chronicle*. But its reverberations were quickly felt across the country at the Connecticut headquarters of Purdue. Years later, lawyers for Fisher said they contacted the pharmaceutical company in 1999, hopeful for its assistance in mounting his defense. Court records also show that expert witnesses working for the state of California also contacted Purdue for information about OxyContin, which, in early 1999, was still a relatively new product on the market.

Fisher's lawyers later said that Purdue officials told them they wouldn't play any part in the case. And Fisher recalled long afterward that a physician associated with the drugmaker explained to him that its executives viewed Purdue as a "conservative" company that liked to avoid controversy.

But like it or not, Fisher's arrest created a crisis within Purdue, and its officials apparently faced a dilemma. The issue: how to treat commissions paid to sales reps based on prescriptions written by doctors under suspicion. In one case, the company in 1999 considered seeking the return of such commissions from a sales rep but subsequently decided not to, one former official familiar with those events subsequently said. Years later, Purdue exectives won't comment on the episode or provide any clarification about it.

The case of Frank Fisher would set the tone for the type of problems involving OxyContin that were emerging in 1999, and newspaper reports were by no means the only way such information was getting to Purdue.

Purdue's six-hundred-person-strong sales force equaled the total number of diversion investigators employed by the DEA, a workforce that was supposed to keep tabs on hundreds of prescription drugs as well as chemicals used to make illicit substance like methamphetamine. But by 1999, Purdue was dedicating about 75 percent of its sales force to promoting OxyContin, and some reps, along with selling the painkiller, gathered information about the drug and funneled it back to their superiors.

It was such a mission that brought two Purdue sales reps in the spring of 1999 to offices of the *Weirton Daily Times*. A physician at a local hospital, the Weirton Medical Center, had alerted William Beatty, the longtime narcotics investigator, that he suspected that drug abusers were coming there from nearby cities such as Pittsburgh to con OxyContin prescriptions from physicians at the hospital's pain clinic. That same spring, after the *Weirton Daily Times* articles appeared, a Purdue official giving a pain management talk at Weirton Medical was even confronted by a doctor there about overdoses caused by the painkiller, said one person who attended that meeting.

Beatty would later recall speaking that spring to the physician who headed the pain clinic and urging him to limit his prescribing. He also said he gave doctors at the hospital a demonstration of how easy it was to defeat OxyContin. "What I did was to go in and show them how to scrape the plastic coating off," Beatty said. "I cooked an OxyContin down for them. It took three or four minutes."

Just how many officials within Purdue learned about events in Weirton and got copies of the article from the *Weirton Daily Times* is anyone's guess. But one thing is known: William Beatty would later say that no one from the company ever called him.

While some people were shooting up OxyContin in 1999, others were abusing the painkiller in the same easy way as Lindsay Myers and her friends. Instead of taking it whole, they crushed a tablet by chewing it up with their teeth and then swallowed or snorted the powder.

In mid-1999, one Purdue sales rep began to file memos about a doctor who said that his patients were chewing Oxy-Contin. As fate would have it, the physician she was calling on was Dr. Richard Norton of Duffield, Virginia, a small town just twenty miles east of Art Van Zee's clinic in St. Charles. Van Zee, Larry Lavender, and Greg Stewart, the druggist, had all come to believe that Norton was prescribing OxyContin to problem patients. But Norton himself, documents suggest, was fast growing wary of the drug.

Norton's comments were captured at the time by the Purdue sales rep in the area, Kimberly Keith. Each time a Purdue sales rep such as Keith visited a physician, she or he generated a so-called call report. These electronic memos, which are used by other drug companies too, are intended to memorialize any issues that arise during a rep's visit with a physician and also to incorporate the rep's ideas about what sales techniques might be used to increase a doctor's prescribing.

Keith's territory covered southwestern Virginia, and she called on both Art Van Zee and area pharmacists such as Greg Stewart. Indeed, Stewart would later recall that Keith was the Purdue sales rep who had initially assured him that OxyContin was less prone to abuse than other narcotics. Copies of call reports indicate that she started seeing Richard Norton in early 1998, and her early memos do not, in fact, reflect any problems with the drug.

But by mid-1999, red flags were appearing in her call reports, which were hastily written in shorthand and contained abbreviations such as "PATS" for patients. For example, Keith wrote after a visit to Norton on July 2:

SAID PATS NOT DOING SO WELL BCAUSE CHEWING OXY ETC, UPSET THAT CAN BREAK TABLET DOWN NOT THAT THEY HAVE FIGURED OUT HOW TO DO IT. DISUCSSED [sic] GIVING IT TO THE RIGHT PATIENTS WOULDN'T BE A CONCERN.

Two weeks later, on July 19, Keith filed another call report reflecting Norton's comments during a follow-up visit. It read:

SAID VERY DISAPPOINTED THAT PURDUE DOESN'T MAKE A CHEMICAL DELIVERY VS A MECHANICAL. ASKED WHY, BCAUSE PATS ARE

CHEWING OXYCONTIN AND GETTING A RUSH.
NOT SEEING LOT OF PATIENTS WITH NECROSIS
[from hypodermic injection]. SAID WAS GOING TO MS
CONTIN BCAUSE DIDN'T SEEM TO GET THE BUZZ
OR EURPHOIA LIKE WITH OXYCONTIN, NEED TO
DISCUSS NEXT TIME.

Keith's subsequent reports were terse and less illuminating.

Norton soon had other problems unrelated to his patients.
In late 2000 he was convicted and sent to prison on federal
fraud charges related to a kickback scheme involving health
care payments. Years later, while still imprisoned, he insisted
that he had been framed by federal officials; he also unleashed
a bitter barrage of claims against Purdue officials, Art Van Zee,
and Greg Stewart.

William Beatty of Weirton, West Virginia, wasn't the only
public official to issue a warning about OxyContin back in
1999. That August the local prosecutor's office of Cambria
County, in southwestern Pennsylvania, sent out an alert to local
doctors.

"A number of disturbing trends in the illegal use of pharmaceutical drugs have come to light in recent days that have
law enforcement in the area alarmed," read the bulletin written
by Ron Portash, the detective who headed the county's Pharmaceutical Enforcement Program. Those trends, Portash continued, included the growing abuse of Ultram, the non-narcotic

painkiller made by Ortho-McNeil. But in his alert, Portash quickly turned to Purdue's efforts to use timed-release formulations as a way to reduce narcotics abuse.

"Drug researchers have been taking this into consideration when designing the new wave of pain killers to hit the market," the prosecutor's office bulletin read. "Of these new pharmaceutical drugs, oxycontin [*sic*] and MS Contin have found a niche in the illegal recreational drug use setting. Pharmaceutical drug abusers have found a way to circumvent the oral administration to negate the long-lasting effect of the drugs, thus producing a 'speed' type of high from the drugs. The local street price runs from $30–$60 per pill."

It's impossible to say who within Purdue received such information in 1999, or what they made of it. But the company's concerns might have been deepening because that September it hired David Haddox, the physician who would soon emerge as its point person on OxyContin. From then on, Haddox publicly defended every action taken by Purdue. But just before joining the drugmaker, he had also written an article in which he warned that efforts to create better pain care might also have a boomerang effect as doctors, facing increasing demands from patients and peer pressure, overprescribed narcotics.

In the December 1998 issue of the *Journal of Law, Medicine and Ethics*, a small publication that often reflected the views of narcotics advocates, Haddox and a coauthor, Dr. Gerald Aronoff, wrote that the growing use of strong narcotics, while medically justified, carried significant risks. One was that pain patients, who were suitable candidates for physical therapy or other types of non-pharmacological treatments, might demand pills instead because taking them was easier than showing up for therapy.

But Haddox and Aronoff pointed to a potentially bigger problem. At the urging of narcotics advocates, many states had adopted so-called Intractable Pain Treatment Acts, guidelines or laws that allowed physicians to prescribe large amounts of opioids if medically justified for severe pain without fear of legal or licensing consequences. The problem, as Haddox and Aronoff saw it, was that those states hadn't made any recommendations about how physicians should be educated about the pharmacology of these powerful drugs so that they would know how and when to best use them.

"With the increased amount of attention these policy changes have received in medical media, it is likely that many physicians who were, heretofore, reluctant to prescribe opioids, now feel it is incumbent to do so," the two men wrote. "Therefore, practitioners who were unfamiliar with their use may begin using them more liberally and may contribute to increased diversion or create complications that could otherwise be foreseen and prevented."

In the fall of 1999, less than a year later, Haddox was working for Purdue. And right about that same time, Dr. Frank Fisher, the California doctor who had been arrested that February, said he called Haddox to complain that one of the company's speakers was misrepresenting OxyContin's resistance to abuse.

A few months earlier, in July, Fisher had been released from jail after four months of imprisonment when the murder charges against him were thrown out or reduced to manslaughter and his bail had been dramatically reduced. Fisher, as he awaited his trial's start, spent much of his time working with his defense lawyers. But he also kept up on pain management issues and remained a strong believer in OxyContin, despite his travails.

Fisher would recall that not long after his release from jail he attended a presentation about pain management at an area hospital that was sponsored by Purdue. He said he was stunned to hear the speaker repeatedly insist that the painkiller couldn't be abused because of its timed-release packaging.

"All the nurses there were laughing about it," Fisher remembered.

Fisher said that the incident had upset him so much that he phoned Purdue's headquarters, where his call was directed to Haddox. He said he recounted the speakers' remarks to Haddox, whom he had never met though knew by reputation. "David, you know that what your lecturers are telling people isn't true," Fisher recalled telling the Purdue medical director.

Fisher described Haddox as sounding very concerned, adding that he asked the physician for the speakers' name and other information about the event. Fisher never knew how his complaint was addressed because he said he never heard back from Haddox.

Before 1999 ended, Purdue would get more bad news about OxyContin from yet another part of the country. The company was alerted about a physician in Florida whose troubles would deepen when he was convicted in 2002 of manslaughter in connection with the deaths of four patients from drug overdoses involving oxycodone. It was news that made national headlines.

The doctor's name was James F. Graves. During the course of his trial it came out that his waiting room was often filled with "people who appeared to be stoned" and that many of Graves' patients had been referred to him by friends rather than physicians. While those patients who died of overdoses had histories of drug abuse, the parents of some of Graves' patients pleaded with him not to prescribe their children more drugs.

"Word spread that he was the go-to doctor," Russell Edgar, a Florida assistant district attorney, told a jury during Graves' trial. "He's no different than a drug dealer."

Purdue had started hearing complaints about Graves, who was prescribing large quantities of OxyContin in 1999, from Leon V. Dulion, the sales rep whose territory covered Graves' practice. Graves, a former Navy doctor, had bounced from job to job before finally opening an office in Pace, Florida, a small town near the city of Pensacola in the state's panhandle section.

Though Graves didn't have any special pain training, his small office increasingly attracted those complaining of pain. For them, he prescribed a mix of medications that local pharmacists soon dubbed the "Graves cocktail." It included painkillers like OxyContin and Lortab as well as the tranquilizer Xanax.

Leon Dulion first called on Graves in the fall of 1998. The salesman later testified that he described OxyContin's benefits to the physician, including the added safety value of its timed-release system. Dulion, a longtime Purdue employee, said he gave the physician copies of material deemed helpful in deterring drug abuse, including a so-called pain contract. A pain contract is essentially an agreement that a patient signs in which he or she promises not to seek narcotics from anyone other than the doctor treating them.

By mid-1999, however, Dulion was starting to hear complaints from area pharmacists that Graves was inappropriately prescribing OxyContin, primarily the 40-milligram- and 80-milligram-strength tablets. Some area drugstores even began refusing to fill his prescriptions. Dulion, who reported back to his superiors, told druggists what he later said Graves had told him—that the high dosages were necessary because the type of pain his patients were experiencing was severe and difficult to treat.

But soon, Dulion had a separate set of concerns about Graves and they centered on whether the physician was giving away free supplies of OxyContin in exchange for money. Graves' scheme was apparently taking advantage of the roundabout way that Purdue used to get free samples of its narcotic into the hands of patients.

Within the pharmaceutical industry, it is standard practice for sales reps to drop off small free sample packets of a new drug as a way to encourage physicians to prescribe the medication to their patients. But sales reps for narcotics makers can't do that because of DEA regulations. Those rules require that everyone who handles such drugs have a permit and that all transfers of narcotics be recorded, a process that makes the distribution of samples by sales reps a practical impossibility.

But pharmaceutical companies have found a perfectly legal way to get around that roadblock. In Purdue's case, company sales reps annually distributed thousands of coupons to doctors, each one good for either a free seven-day or free thirty-day trial supply of OxyContin. A physician prescribing OxyContin would give a coupon to a patient who then took it to a drugstore and got the painkiller for free. In internal budgets, Purdue put the annual cost of its giveaway program at $4 million.

Dulion would later tell prosecutors that in the first few months of 1999 he received thirty such coupons and gave six of them to Graves, each one good for a free thirty-day supply of the painkiller. But he discovered in late 1999 that Graves may have been trying to get something back in return. By then, Dulion's sales duties had shifted and he no longer called on the Pace doctor. But in visiting the office of another area physician, Dulion got involved in a conversation that became seared into his memory. He would also tell prosecutors that he reported the incident back to his superiors.

The Purdue rep said that when he arrived at the physician's office, two patients—a man and a woman—were discussing the types of drugs that were available for sale on the street. Soon their conversation turned to how the DEA was investigating a doctor in Pace and how that physician would probably soon be shut down. The woman explained how that physician, Dr. Graves, used to give out a coupon "that would get you all your OxyContin for free" if you agreed to sign up for a long-distance telephone service offered through a company called Excel. Her comments, Dulion told prosecutors, hit a chord with him; he knew that Graves ran a side business selling telephone services because the Purdue rep had purchased some from him.

Dulion then testified that the woman looked over at him and said, "I hope I didn't offend you."

He said he then identified himself as an OxyContin sales rep.

"Oh, I'm so sorry," the woman told Dulion. "OxyContin is an excellent medication. I'm a recovering addict."

Dulion told the woman that he had happened to overhear her and her friend discussing street drugs. He said that he had always understood that hydrocodone-containing drugs like Vicodin and Lortab were the most widely abused painkillers.

The woman told him he was wrong, at least where the streets of Pensacola were concerned. "On the street the number one abused drug is crack cocaine, which they call the devil's dick, followed by OxyContin, which they refer to as the devil's balls."

It was only a few months later that Jay McCloskey issued his alert to Maine doctors. Over time, company executives would slowly roll out a series of responses to the drug's growing abuse that would culminate more than fifteen months later with their decision to drop the claim that OxyContin was less attractive as a drug of abuse. That move followed but by a few months intense media publicity about the drug's problems.

It seemed that during 2000, the year when the OxyContin problem was taking even greater hold, there appeared to be two Purdues. While David Haddox and others were assigned the job of addressing the issue of misuse, the company's marketing machine careened ahead as though on a separate track. For example, field reps received weekly messages from top marketing officials through the company's voicemail exhorting them to increase sales.

"We are setting new records," a former sales rep remembers one of the messages as saying. "We are blowing away our objectives and our goals."

Just what information, if any, Purdue executives distributed in early 2000 to its sales force about the painkiller's growing abuse is not known. But it may have been little.

Kerry Rowland, a former narcotics detective in Cincinnati, recalled how ten Purdue sales reps descended upon his office soon after an article that described OxyContin's growing abuse in that city appeared in a police department newsletter. The Purdue sales officials all insisted he was wrong.

"They said it really couldn't be abused and it was not being abused and they were concerned about what I had written," he recalled. "I told them I had nothing against Purdue or Oxy-Contin. I didn't care what the drug was. But the fact of the matter was that it was being abused."

In mid-2000, Mark Radcliffe, a Purdue district manager in West Virginia, also counseled a company sales rep about how to remain "Audible Ready" on the issue of street abuse. In that August 2000 memo, in which Radcliffe reviewed the sales rep's performance during some joint visits they had recently made to doctors and pharmacists, he wrote:

You continue to get hammered with pre-1990 attitudes about opioids. Dr. Steinberg shocked me! This Harvard trained physician and expert for medical cases said to you "Do you know how many days it takes to get addicted? Five and then they are addicted!" The pharmacist at Clark's informed us that they are doing "everything they can to slow it down (OxyContin)." Despite these relentless attacks, you've done a good job of remaining "Audible Ready" on the street abuse issue and not letting the "phobics" sell you. Distinguish between iatrogenic addiction (<1% of patients) and substance abusers/diversion (about 10 percent of the population abuse something: weed; cocaine; heroin; alcohol; valium; etc.)

Purdue officials, other than describing July 2001 as the "appropriate" time to drop that claim, have never said why they didn't do so earlier; nor have they ever discussed the reasons they felt the need to make such a claim for OxyContin. They had never done so for MS Contin.

In March 1995, however, top company sales executives such as Michael Friedman had received a marketing report that may have helped set the stage for the events that followed. One of its recommendations was that if Purdue could show that Oxy-Contin posed a lower risk of abuse than traditional immediate-release narcotics, sales of the new painkiller might increase.

Though Purdue executives have said they never ran those specific tests, FDA officials approved a labeling claim for Oxy-

Contin that conveyed just that implication. And in the years that followed it would become a rallying cry for the drug, one that Purdue would cling to. Finally, that claim would be revealed for what it had been—an illusionary signpost along Oxy-Contin's long trail of addiction and death. But by then, six years would have passed and thousands of lives been altered, many of them irrevocably.

Thousands of people were undergoing treatment for drug addiction and not all of them were drug abusers. Pain patients too were part of that mix, people who had innocently gone into their doctors' offices seeking relief from one problem and found themselves saddled with another one, drug abuse or addiction. There was no way of telling how many there were, but one thing was for sure: Purdue was no longer saying that such incidences of iatrogenic addiction were "extremely rare."

Meanwhile, by 2002 the human toll taken by the abuse and misuse of prescription narcotics such as OxyContin had become increasingly alarming. That year, for instance, the *South Florida Sun-Sentinel* reported that its review of medical examiner data had found that nearly four hundred people had died from prescription drug overdoses over a two-year period in just one part of that state, the area in and around the cities of Miami, Fort Lauderdale, and Palm Beach. The vast majority of those deaths involved narcotic painkillers containing oxycodone or hydrocodone, and many of those who had died had been able to obtain large quantities of painkillers from doctors despite documented histories of drug abuse, the paper reported.

A cascade of ripple effects also followed in OxyContin's

wake. During the height of the crisis involving the painkiller, the ranks of methadone clinics were swelled with those abusing the drug. Such programs helped many people reclaim their lives. But the increasing use of methadone also increased supplies of it on the street for sale and that had its own deadly consequences.

Methadone, while a valuable painkiller and addiction maintenance substance, can be lethal, particularly in the hands of inexperienced users. The reasons relate to the nature of the drug; methadone does not produce its high as quickly as heroin or oxycodone and also it lingers in the body for far longer. As a result, inexperienced users or abusers of the drug can make a fatal mistake; eager to get high, they keep taking more methadone, creating a buildup of the drug that can produce a deadly overdose. By mid-2002, states around the country, including many that had experienced high rates of illegal OxyContin use, were reporting sharp increases in the number of methadone-related overdose deaths.

Lindsay Myers was one of the lucky ones. On New Year's Day of 2003, she lay in a hospital room in Johnson City, Tennessee, screaming in pain. A few hours later, her son was born. He was healthy and weighed six pounds and eleven ounces. His first name was Brennon, but Lindsay and Jane started calling him by his middle name, Kyle.

Jane had already realized that she—not Lindsay or her daughter's new boyfriend—would have to take care of Kyle. She had fixed up a part of her bedroom with a crib, a changing table, and toys. Kyle arrived there two days after he was born.

In the desperate weeks before Kyle's birth, Jane and Johnny, at Larry Lavender's urging, had given Lindsay a choice. She could go into a residential treatment program, or they would have her prosecuted for larceny for stealing the family's jewelry.

A few weeks after Kyle was born, Lindsay left for the Hazelden Clinic, the well-known substance abuse treatment facility in Minnesota where celebrities have gone for help. After a successful month there, she left to stay at a halfway house in Phoenix, Arizona. During a telephone call with Jane, Lindsay wondered if maybe things would be better if she didn't come back to Lee County or her boyfriend. Maybe it was time for her and Kyle to start a new life somewhere else.

NEW
BEGINNINGS

THE LIGHT ON THE TELE-
phone answering machine was
flashing when Sister Beth
Davies walked into her office at
the Addiction Education Center
in downtown Pennington Gap.
As soon as she pushed the play-
back button, a woman's cheerful
voice leapt out from the machine.

"Hi, I'm Melissa Karron from
Beverly Enterprises," the woman
said. "We want to donate a
building to you."

Beth was dumbstruck. Then
she raced around the center until
she found Elizabeth Vines and Larry
Lavender so they could hear the message. As they listened to the
tape, the same thought hit them all at the same time.

For years, people who needed intensive, ongoing treatment
for drug addiction had to stay at a center called the Laurels in

Lebanon, Virginia, a town that was a two-hour drive from Pennington Gap. Ever since the nightmare of OxyContin abuse had descended, the three addiction counselors had shared the common dream of having a similar facility nearby. Now, it appeared that with a sudden phone call in the spring of 2002, they were being handed a building that might serve as one.

Beverly Enterprises was a company that operated a large nationwide chain of nursing homes, including one called the Carter Hall Nursing Home on the outskirts of Pennington Gap. The one-story, concrete-block building sat on a four-acre site just off the highway that ran toward Dryden, the town where Art Van Zee and Sue Ella lived. Over the years, Sister Beth had gotten to know lots of people who worked at Carter Hall, and some of them had told her the nursing home would be closing because Beverly Enterprises was about to complete work on a new and bigger facility. Still, no one had talked about the company's plans for the older building.

Sister Beth called the corporate offices of Beverly Enterprises in Fort Smith, Arkansas, and asked to be connected to Melissa Karron.

"Can you explain to me what this is all about?"

The company official told Beth that Beverly Enterprises had a policy of donating its closed buildings to local towns or civic groups. She mentioned that a number of employees at Carter Hall had recommended that it be given to the Addiction Education Center. They saw it as a way of thanking Sister Beth and Elizabeth Vines for all the help they had given to the families of Lee County over the past twenty years, including some of their own.

Sister Beth replied that she was overjoyed by the company's offer but thought that perhaps a bigger group like the Lee Coalition for Health was better suited than the addiction center to take on the project. Beth was told that whatever the community decided was fine with Beverly Enterprises.

Beth quickly called Art Van Zee and told him what was happening.

"You're kidding!" he responded.

"This is real," she insisted. "We have to talk about this."

Two days later, Van Zee, Sister Beth, and the other members of the Lee Coalition for Health met at the hospital to discuss whether to accept the building. Unlike Purdue's offer of $100,000 to the group, Beth and the others didn't feel like they would have to give up something of themselves in return. Still, taking over the fifty-bed facility was a huge responsibility, and some members wondered how or even whether the Coalition could manage it. A lot of costly work needed to be done to convert the nursing home to a treatment center; for one, it would have to be completely remodeled into separate wings for male and female residents.

"If we take this building, we are responsible right away," Sister Beth told the group. And those costs, both short- and long-term, would be significant, she explained. The Coalition would need to immediately start paying for insurance, electricity, and hot water, and it had to hire someone to maintain the facility's grounds. Coalition members like Van Zee and

Sister Beth had never been short of energy, but the group didn't have a regular income and its bank account held only a few hundred dollars.

Still, Van Zee and the others decided to take a chance; in Lee County this kind of opportunity wasn't going to happen again. By the time the Coalition's meeting broke up, everyone had volunteered to take on a job: to check with the electric company, to make sure that the hot water remained on, to find out from Carter Hall's administrator what urgent repair work needed to be done. Sue Ella volunteered to take on the legal work, and soon she was on the telephone with a Beverly Enterprises lawyer on the property's transfer to the Lee Coalition. The group decided to rename the building for its future life as a treatment center. They would call it New Beginnings.

For Larry Lavender, the prospect of the treatment center's opening represented a new start as well. In early 2003 he accepted the job as the center's director and began traveling to conferences and meetings to prepare himself as an administrator. By then, a few local judges had been convinced by Sue Ella and others that some OxyContin abusers would do better in treatment than in jail, and Lavender wanted to make New Beginnings into a place where they could come.

To help pay for the costs of converting the building, the Coalition began holding fund-raisers. They held a $10-a-plate dinner, and on another occasion the group organized a craft fair. Contributions came in from local families, including many like Jane and Johnny Myers who had seen a child's life derailed by OxyContin. Area businesses gave, too: one bank made a contribution of $5,000, and the John Deere distributor donated a lawn mower and a snowplow.

By early 2003 the group had raised about $35,000, although that money was eaten up quickly by remodeling and repair costs that included a new roof for the building. The Coalition estimated that New Beginnings, once opened, would cost more than $150,000 a year to run because they wanted people from throughout coal country to be able to come there for treatment even if they didn't have insurance.

As a result, Art Van Zee was back down in his basement working again. This time, though, he wasn't hammering out letters to OxyContin's maker, Purdue, or to the FDA, but trying to figure out how to do something that he had never tried before: writing applications to federal agencies and foundations for grant money to help fund New Beginnings.

About the same time, Russell Portenoy was sitting in his office at Beth Israel Medical Center in New York, reflecting on the OxyContin episode. The debacle hadn't dented his belief in the medical value of long-acting narcotics, but it had sobered him to the use of arbitrary research to push the cause of better pain care. "It was pseudoscience," he remarked. "I guess I'm going to have always to live with that one."

Portenoy, like many of his colleagues in the pain management movement, was still trying to make sense of what had gone wrong with OxyContin, trying to understand why the drug's problems had become so severe. He suspected, as many others did, that Purdue's aggressive marketing of OxyContin had played a central role; maybe not so much the specific techniques but rather the thrust of the marketing. After all, Portenoy reasoned, no company had ever before promoted such a pure, high-strength Schedule II narcotic to so wide an audience of general practitioners and others untrained in its use.

But he had also begun to wonder whether there was something unique about OxyContin's active ingredient, oxycodone. Purdue executives had repeatedly pointed to MS Contin's low incidence of problems as a leading reason why they had been caught unawares by the size of the recreational appetite for OxyContin. But morphine and oxycodone, while belonging to the same class of drugs, were different substances with their own unique properties.

Some researchers believed that oxycodone might give a better high. One of them was James Zacny of the University of Chicago. For years, Zacny had conducted experiments with student volunteers to determine the effects that various opioids had on physical skills like reaction time to stimuli and hand-eye coordination. Zacny also tried to determine whether his volunteers experienced a sense of euphoria.

Zacny's experiments with morphine in healthy students yielded similar results to those seen by Russell Portenoy and Kathleen Foley among cancer sufferers at Memorial Sloan-Kettering. Portenoy and Foley had reported that cancer patients rarely became euphoric after taking morphine, and Zacny's students didn't have dramatically different reactions. Some other widely used narcotics, including hydrocodone, the active ingredient in drugs like Vicodin, also produced some euphoria among student volunteers. But when Zacny tested oxycodone on volunteers, he got different results; a number of students reported experiencing euphoria and pleasant body sensations. Some of them also said they'd use the drug again.

"It sort of raised my eyebrows," Zacny remembered.

Zacny said that his test population was too small to draw any conclusions from it, but he expects to continue exploring whether oxycodone holds a special lure. Lindsay Myers would know. She and Ray tried MS Contin. Lindsay and Ray crushed up the morphine pills and snorted them just as they would have done with an Oxy.

"We didn't get a buzz from it," Lindsay remembered. "We didn't like it at all."

By early 2003, despite the celebratory communiqués dispatched from company headquarters every time a lawsuit against it was dismissed, other lawsuits filed against Purdue, including those from people claiming to have become addicted to OxyContin as a result of pain treatment, had moved forward. The dismissals had likely been just the initial skirmishes in a legal battle over the painkiller that probably would stretch out for years, one whose ultimate resolution was by no means clear.

Meanwhile, congressional investigators had decided to again look at OxyContin. The House Energy and Commerce Committee, which was chaired by Representative W. J. "Billy" Tauzin of Louisiana, ordered Purdue to provide it with all depositions given by company sales reps in connection with litigation involving OxyContin. The committee also wanted information on how Purdue had compensated its sales force. Separately, Purdue officials received a request for documents from a U.S. attorney in Virginia, though the focus of that investigation wasn't clear.

The renewed congressional interest in the drugmaker apparently had been piqued by its efforts to again win FDA approval for its timed-release version of the painkiller Dilaudid, a drug that Purdue had been selling in Canada for several years under the brand name Palladone. DEA officials had expressed concerns to members of Tauzin's committee that the abuse of Palladone could exceed that of OxyContin. While that was speculation, Tauzin's committee decided it wanted data that compared hydromorphone, the active ingredient in both Dilaudid and Palladone, to oxycodone in terms of its potential for abuse and addiction. As a result, the FDA's review of Palladone, which some observers had believed was poised to win agency approval in early 2003, appeared to slow.

Meanwhile, despite the extensive interaction between Purdue executives and the FDA since mid-2001, the company had again run into trouble with the agency. In November 2002, the *Journal of the American Medical Association* carried a full-page ad for OxyContin that bore the headline "There Can Be Life With Relief." The ad's photograph portrayed a seemingly happy, healthy-looking man fly-fishing in a rural stream in the company of a young boy who might have been his grandchild.

The lifestyle ad may have been the product of a growing concern among Purdue sales officials that they were losing the battle for a vital category of pain patients. An internal Purdue report written in 2001 noted, for instance, that the Janssen division of Johnson & Johnson had been increasingly promoting its fentanyl-containing pain patch, Duragesic, for "moderate-to-moderately severe" pain, or the same patients that Purdue was seeking for OxyContin.

But Purdue executives, a company document noted, were worried about claims that Janssen could make for Duragesic that OxyContin couldn't match.

"Janssen has been stressing decreased side effects, especially constipation, as well as patient quality of life, as supported by patient rating compared to sustained-released morphine," the budget document stated. "We do not have such data to support OxyContin promotion. . . . In addition, Janssen had been using the 'life uninterrupted' message in promotion of Duragesic for non-cancer pain, stressing that Duragesic 'helps patients think less about their pain.' This is a competitive advantage based on our inability to make any quality of life claims."

A part of Purdue's marketing strategy for OxyContin in 2002 would stress its value in "improving the quality of life, mood and sleep," the same document noted. And the upbeat November ad in the *Journal of the American Medical Association* may well have been a part of that campaign.

Whatever the case, Purdue's ad in *JAMA* was seen not only by thousands of doctors but by FDA officials too. The agency soon sent the company a seven-page warning letter that severely rebuked it for the ad as well as a similar one that had run in the same publication a month earlier. The agency annually sends out hundreds of similar so-called warning letters alerting companies that the agency believes they are violating federal regulations. For example, Purdue had withdrawn an OxyContin ad in 2000 after FDA officials sent company executives a warning letter saying thy believed the ad implied that OxyContin could be used to treat arthritis patients without trying milder drugs first.

However, the more recent warning letter employed unusually harsh language. It was written by Thomas W. Abrams, the director of the FDA's division of Drug Marketing, Advertising and Communications, and in his letter Abrams noted that Purdue, among other things, hadn't even put OxyContin's black-box warning on the ad's cheerful-looking cover page. Instead it appeared on the backside of the ad, along with fine-print information about the painkiller's uses and risks.

A part of Abrams' letter, which was addressed to Michael Friedman, stated:

> Neither one of your ads presents in the body of the advertisements any information from the boxed warning discussing OxyContin's potential for abuse and the related considerations when prescribing the drug. Neither one of your ads presents in the body of the advertisements any information from the boxed warning disclosing that the drug can be fatal if taken by certain patients or under certain conditions. It is particularly disturbing that your November Ad would tout "Life With Relief" yet fail to warn that patients can die from taking OxyContin.

Despite everything that had occurred over the past two years—
the huge upsurge involving OxyContin's abuse and the damage
created to both young people and the interests of pain patients—Purdue, Abrams effectively charged, was still pushing
the drug's marketing envelope by understating its dangers and
promoting OxyContin for uses for which it hadn't been approved. He wrote:

> Your advertisements thus grossly overstate the safety of
> OxyContin by not referring in the body of the advertisements to
> serious, potentially fatal risks associated with OxyContin,
> thereby potentially leading to prescribing of the product based
> on inadequate consideration of the risk. In addition, your
> journal advertisements fail to present in the body of the
> advertisements critical information regarding limitations on the
> indicated use of OxyContin, thereby promoting OxyContin for
> a much broader range of patients with pain than are
> appropriate for the drug. The combination in these
> advertisements of suggesting such a broad use of this drug to
> treat pain without disclosing the potential for abuse with the
> drug and the serious, potentially fatal risks associated with its
> use, is especially egregious and alarming in its potential impact
> on the public health.

Purdue executives quickly announced that OxyContin's black-
box warning would appear on all future ads for the painkiller.
As to why they had omitted it on the upbeat fly-fishing scene in

the *Journal of the American Medical Association* ad, it had all
been the result, they insisted, of a "misunderstanding."

In the late winter of 2003, a number of people whose lives had
become entwined with OxyContin arrived for a conference at
a building in midtown Manhattan, a few blocks away from
Grand Central Station. The building contained the offices of the
National Center on Addiction and Substance Abuse, a think
tank associated with Columbia University. The group had been
founded in the early 1990s by Joseph A. Califano Jr., secretary
of the Department of Health, Education, and Welfare during
the administration of President Jimmy Carter. Ever since, it has
conducted studies on a range of social issues such as teenage
drinking, drug use, and sexual behavior.

Purdue executives had approached the group and offered it
$1 million to help underwrite a study about pain treatment and
the abuse of prescription narcotics. Califano's group was initially leery of accepting the drugmaker's funds but agreed to do
so after the drug company's executives said they wouldn't seek
any editorial control over their report.

Work on that report was still under way in February 2003
when the organization, which regularly hosted conferences,
held one at its Manhattan headquarters about prescription drug
abuse and pain treatment. The biggest single presence at the
conference, which attracted about a hundred people, was
Purdue. As was its frequent practice, the drugmaker had again

flooded the zone. David Haddox was there as an invited speaker, and Robin Hogen, the drugmaker's spokesperson, sat in the audience along with at least four other Purdue employees. Also on the roster of those attending the meeting were the names of five lawyers from King & Spalding, the firm that Purdue had hired to organize its defense against OxyContin-related lawsuits. It wasn't clear from the program whether Purdue was paying them each the common law firm billing rate of $400 an hour to attend the day-long conference, or if the company had qualified for a discounted group rate.

A number of panels of experts spoke at the conference on topics such as the physiology of drug addiction, the ethics of pharmaceutical marketing, and the training of doctors in the treatment of pain. The day's last expert panel was titled "Diversion: Medical Judgment and the Judgment of Medicine"; its members included Laura Nagel, the head of the DEA's diversion office, and David Haddox.

Two years had passed now since Nagel had taken her job and walked wide-eyed into the storm that was OxyContin. Her knowledge of the legal narcotics industry was now better attuned and she had started working closely with some drugmakers on their plans to monitor abuse of their products.

Nagel hadn't initially wanted to attend the meeting at the National Center on Addiction and Substance Abuse. It wasn't that she had anything against the group, but Nagel continued to be offended by Purdue's constant spreading of its money and preferred to avoid those who took it.

In her remarks to the conference that February day, Nagel repeated the agency's now-familiar position that the DEA had no intention of cutting off the supply of needed narcotics to pain patients. It was a comment that drew skeptical responses from some audience members who still continued to view the agency as more interested in busting doctors that bettering pain care.

Haddox carried Purdue's flag. Throughout the meeting he responded to questions about OxyContin by putting the company's best foot forward. He repeatedly cited all the programs the drugmaker had initiated to combat prescription drug abuse. He described the recent dispute with the FDA over the company's ads for OxyContin as a "misunderstanding." It seemed that for much of the day he was reading from a script carefully vetted by teams of lawyers and public relations consultants.

The Purdue medical director also used the meeting to announce some of the "findings" of a Purdue-funded study of medical examiner reports of drug overdose deaths, a survey that Purdue had undertaken in response to the DEA's effort. Not surprisingly, Haddox's remarks, as well as a press release about the study, sought to minimize OxyContin's involvement in the death reports. For instance, the press release trumpeted the fact that only thirty of the one thousand deaths reviewed as part of Purdue's study involved oxycodone alone. And of those deaths, an even tinier fraction, just twelve cases, were instances in which OxyContin was identified as the source of the oxycodone involved.

It could hardly have been news to toxicologists, or to

Haddox, for that matter, that the vast majority of people who died in OxyContin-related overdoses didn't just have oxycodone in their systems. For example, a 2001 analysis of medical examiner data collected through DAWN, the hospital emergency room system, found that 92 percent of prescription narcotic deaths involved multiple drugs rather than a single substance.

But when those rare cases involving a single substance were set aside, the percentage of overdose deaths in which Purdue's painkiller may have played a part was stunning, even by the drugmaker's reckoning. For instance, the Purdue-funded study, using criteria similar to the DEA's, definitively identified Oxy-Contin as the source of the oxycodone detected in about 20 percent of one thousand overdose deaths reviewed, virtually the exact percentage found by Dave Gauvin, the agency official. Purdue's consultants also found a high percentage of cases in which oxycodone but not aspirin or acetaminophen had been found, the cases that DEA had cited as "OxyContin-likely." Those consultants, however, said they couldn't rule out oxycodone-containing combination painkillers like Percocet in such deaths because toxicological tests to identify aspirin or acetaminophen weren't reliable.

As the day-long meeting in New York came to a close, David Haddox was asked by a panel's moderator, George Strait, a former television news reporter, if he believed that Purdue had made any mistakes in its handling of the Oxy-Contin episode. Haddox's response was immediate and unequivocal.

"I don't think we did anything wrong," he replied.

Months later, Haddox's words would still be ringing in Laura Nagel's ears.

In the summer of 2003, Lindsay Myers came back to Pennington Gap to visit her son Kyle, and her parents. Her recovery appeared to be going well, but soon after getting back to town she realized that she didn't want to stay. She didn't want to see her old boyfriend, Kyle's father. She also decided that she couldn't take care of Kyle, for now at least. Back in Phoenix she had a job waiting for her as a clerk in a hotel and she was going to counseling meetings just about every night. She wanted to start college in the fall. Being a single mom on top of it all just would be too much.

Johnny agreed to drive her back to Arizona in her Jeep. Jane didn't believe she'd really go but she and Johnny were prepared to legally adopt Kyle. As Lindsay was packing up her things, Jane kept waiting for the moment when her daughter would announce that she had changed her mind. She even listened as Lindsay and Johnny started down the hill in the Jeep, expecting to hear it stop. It didn't.

CHAPTER THIRTEEN

THE PAIN INDUSTRY

BY THE CLOSE OF 2002, the red-hot fire that was Oxy-Contin had cooled in places like Lee County, although scattered problems continued to flare up elsewhere. Newspapers in Michigan, Wisconsin, and even the Canadian province of Nova Scotia published reports about local abuse, and pharmacies in some areas, including Boston, remained the targets of robbers. A growing number of drugstores had decided to stop carrying the drug, and in a bid to halt the trend, Purdue announced in late 2002 that it would replace any OxyContin taken by thieves. It was a reasonable offer, though one that might not reassure a pharmacist worried about having a gun pointed at his head.

Street supplies of the drug had dried up as a result of efforts by law enforcement officials, Purdue, and the decision by doctors to prescribe the medication more selectively. OxyContin remained approved for use by the FDA and there was a continuing legitimate need for it; in 2002, despite all the troubles surrounding the painkiller, its sales exceeded $1 billion. Still, the years of the painkiller's extraordinary growth had ended, and along with them the days of heady bonuses for Purdue sales reps. Some reps had left the company to seek better opportunities elsewhere; a few would say later they grew tired of being asked about the drug's abuse by doctors, by pharmacists, by friends, and even by neighbors as if they were somehow responsible for what had happened. Purdue executives did their best to buck up the spirits of those who remained. In 2002, for example, it held a regional sales conference for OxyContin reps working the southeastern United States that had as its rallying motto "Champions despite Uncommon Adversity."

The ultimate tragedy of the OxyContin episode was that it didn't have to happen; at least not in the way it unfolded. But pain management advocates, drug company executives, regulators, and law enforcement officials blindly marched forward, venturing ever deeper into one of medicine's most chaotic realms, the pain industry—an industry that, much like pain itself, defies simple definition or description. Its most visible and respected members, physicians such as Russell Portenoy, are compassionate professionals who use powerful drugs and complementary techniques to help those whose lives are tormented by pain. But the ranks of these highly skilled specialists are thin,

sad testimony to the failure of the medical establishment to provide adequate training in pain treatment for decades.

The OxyContin fiasco may change that. Today, serious pain
is still often treated by doctors who, while well intentioned,
often don't have the time or skills to both properly assess pain
and identify patients most likely to abuse drugs. Substance
abuse and drug addiction are not rare artifacts of medical treatment—they are very real side effects of narcotics and other
drugs. Downplaying those risks, as narcotics advocates and
drug companies are prone to do, is a prescription for disaster;
one need only look at OxyContin.

That doesn't mean that OxyContin and other powerful narcotics shouldn't be used. The lives of untold numbers of people
suffering from severe pain have been improved by such medications. While the risks of abuse and addiction posed by narcotics to pain patients are still unknown, even a tangible level
of risk is an acceptable one for such patients given the prospects
of relief from constant anguish.

But that level of uncertainty means that the use of drugs like
OxyContin should be reserved for serious cases, not doled out
indiscriminately by doctors or marketed by companies as re-
placements for weaker, less-abusable drugs. Such drugs were always intended as a treatment of last resort, originally for a
small fraction of chronic pain patients for whom all other ther-
apies had failed—a special "subpopulation," as Russell
Portenoy called the group. While drug companies like Purdue
and pain management advocates bandy about the figure that 50
million Americans suffer from chronic pain, it is a figure that,

along with lacking any scientific credibility, is a misleading one. Many pain patients could benefit from non-pharmacological treatments like physical therapy. The trouble is that selling pills—in this case, narcotics—is where the money is.

It was somewhere around the mid-1990s, as the height of the pain management movement and the marketing of Oxy-Contin converged, that the boundary lines between "severe" pain and "moderate" pain, "chronic" pain and "acute" pain, blurred and became lost. A drug once reserved as a last line of treatment for the most severe pain cases was promoted as a treatment to be used on medicine's front lines for a wide range of general and transient pain problems. It is hard to believe, despite Purdue's arguments to the contrary, that this broadening availability of OxyContin, a drug classified as the most potentially addicting medication legally available, along with the minimizing of its abuse potential, did not play a crucial role in setting the stage for the disaster that followed.

Those who work for manufacturers such as Purdue can justifiably take pride in their efforts to develop medications to improve patients' lives. But in their zeal to defend themselves and their company, Purdue executives like Michael Friedman, Howard Udell, and David Haddox frequently draped themselves in a mantle of righteousness, suggesting in a variety of ways that the business of selling pain pills is somehow on a par with missionary work.

In fact, the pain business can be as ruthless as any other. In

March 2001, the very month when OxyContin's abuse burst into public view in the United States, British regulators handed down a little-noticed decision against Purdue's sister company, Napp Pharmaceuticals. The ruling found that the British arm of the Sackler pharmaceutical empire had grabbed far more than its fair share of the profits of pain. Regulators in England said that Napp had acted as a financial predator, stifling competition in order to maintain excessive prices and profits for its timed-release, morphine-based painkiller MST, the same drug sold as MS Contin in the United States.

In early 2001 the Office of the Director of Fair Trading in London ordered Napp to pay a fine of $4.57 million, which included an added fine because regulators found that the company continued its predatory pricing scheme even while it was aware that it was under investigation. Napp executives denied any wrongdoing, but an appeals commission subsequently upheld the original ruling, though it reduced Napp's fine by about $1.5 million.

There is no reason to believe that Purdue executives ever foresaw the catastrophe that OxyContin would create. They simply hoped like every other pharmaceutical maker to profit. Similar disasters have befallen other drugmakers and every pharmaceutical company lives with the dread that it might be next.

Still, companies react to misfortune in their own unique ways. And if there was a thread to actions of Purdue executives, it was this: they seemed unable or unwilling to take dramatic action until long after circumstances or adverse publicity had forced their hand. The company did eventually roll out an impressive array of programs and policies aimed at reducing the painkiller's misprescription and abuse—but by then it was far too late.

The actions eventually put into place by Purdue might not have only limited the abuse of OxyContin, but such programs, if adopted by other drugmakers, could help prevent similar tragedies from occurring. For example, one outgrowth of Purdue's negotiations with FDA officials in 2001 was the creation of a panel of consultants to advise the company on drug abuse–related issues. The group's job was to set up a system to provide the company with real-time information about trends involving the abuse of prescription narcotics, including Oxy-Contin. Such an approach is particularly valuable because most existing reporting systems, such as DAWN's emergency room data, are limited in scope or lack timeliness.

While Purdue's creation of the panel, which it dubbed RADARS, was important, it was by no means novel. In fact, in the very year that OxyContin's sale was approved, the Ortho-McNeil division of Johnson & Johnson put into place a monitoring system that, if used by Purdue from the beginning to track OxyContin, might well have reduced its abuse. The drug involved was Ultram, the non-narcotic painkiller that Purdue executives planned to compete against, according to company marketing documents. Prior to its sale, Ortho-McNeil argued to the FDA in 1995 that it should be permitted to sell Ultram as an "unscheduled" drug—that is, one not placed in a controlled substance category—because its active ingredient, tramadol, had long been used in Europe with little evidence of problems.

FDA officials were leery, however, so Ortho-McNeil executives presented the agency with a plan that year that called for the creation of an extensive early warning system to alert the company to signs of Ultram abuse, as well as to quantify that abuse in terms of prescriptions written for the drug. To do so, the company funded the creation of an independent panel of addiction experts who developed an extensive monitoring strategy. The group forged links, for example, with 110 drug abuse and methadone treatment centers around the country that were paid to monitor their patients for Ultram misuse and report their findings back to the panel every three months. Any abuse incidents were then followed up by the team for possible trends. The group also regularly eavesdropped on an increasingly popular form of communication during the 1990s, Internet chat rooms, to see if drug abusers were swapping tips about Ultram. In just a few years, OxyContin would be a hot topic in such chat rooms.

In addition to creating a surveillance system, the same panel reviewed the scientific accuracy of the promotional material used by Ortho-McNeil to market Ultram and lectured sales reps about the painkiller's abuse potential. Panel members also talked to doctors to make sure that the company's sales reps were clearly presenting that information.

Based on that monitoring and the number of prescriptions

being written for Ultram, Ortho-McNeil officials were able to say with some certainty that the rate at which Ultram was being abused was low. When the OxyContin problem erupted, Purdue executives could only guess. Tellingly, years later, when the drugmaker formed RADARS, it retained every consultant hired in 1995 by Ortho-McNeil to monitor Ultram's misuse.

Illegal pill mills, much like prescription drug abuse, existed long before the first tablet of OxyContin tumbled over Purdue's production line. But the virulence of the OxyContin episode threw a spotlight on an aspect of the pain industry that pharmaceutical manufacturers prefer not to confront—the profits they derive from the inappropriate or illegal prescription of their drugs and what they can do about it.

The marketing of OxyContin inadvertently stirred up the pain industry's dark side, its dank corners that are called home by physicians who are medicine's outcasts or even criminals in white coats. For them, medications such as OxyContin aren't healing tools but instruments of barter, sought-after commodities in a black marketplace where prescriptions are traded for cash.

By early 2003 the list of doctors going to jail for illegally prescribing OxyContin and other controlled substances was still growing. Some of those already serving time, like Ali Sawaf of Kentucky and James Graves of Florida, continued to proclaim their innocence. In mid-2003, Dr. Frank Fisher was still a free man; the previous December, California prosecutors had dropped the charges against him and the owners of the Shasta Pharmacy on the eve of their trial, although they said they planned to refile them. Fisher wasn't practicing, but he maintained his innocence.

It would be unrealistic to expect executives of Purdue or any drug company to play cop. They don't get paid or promoted based on the number of arrests but on the profits they make, which adds up to the number of pills the company sells. In fact, many drug company executives might have responded exactly as Purdue's Michael Friedman did in mid-2001 when asked by congressional investigators why the company hadn't looked into the activities of Dr. Paolino, the operator of the OxyContin pill mill in Bensalem, Pennsylvania. As Friedman told lawmakers, Purdue didn't "measure or assess" how a doctor practiced based on his or her prescribing volume.

But the reality is that pharmaceutical companies typically know a lot more than the cops do about the quality and nature of a physician's practice. They spend millions of dollars to buy data from firms such as IMS Health that provide them with exquisitely detailed information that can point to doctors like Paolino who are bad apples. Equally important, they get eyewitness reports on a regular basis from sales reps who visit with physicians.

Should they choose, drug companies could share their suspicions with law enforcement. But even if they don't wish to take that road, there is another option available to them: they could order their sales reps to avoid certain physicians or adopt policies that encourage them to do so. The problem, however, is that such actions conflict with the very rewards and incentives that drugmakers use to motivate both company executives and sales reps.

Consider the case of a pain clinic in Myrtle Beach, South Carolina. It was hardly a secret in the oceanfront resort town that a certain clinic, Comprehensive Care and Pain Management, was a likely trouble spot. In 2000, DEA diversion agents raided Comprehensive Care as part of an investigation into the prescribing practices of physicians working there, seizing three thousand patient files. Drugstore owners working both in Myrtle Beach and in towns as far as a hundred miles away began telling Purdue sales reps that suspicious "patients" were traveling by the carload to Comprehensive Care to get Oxy-Contin prescriptions there. The scene outside the clinic was also hardly reassuring; business owners who shared the same strip mall with the pain clinic said that on many days a line of fifteen to twenty customers stood outside its door for a spot in a packed waiting room. Dozens of cars, many of them with out-of-state license plates, jammed the mall's parking lot from morning to night.

The local Purdue sales rep, Eric Wilson, frequently visited Comprehensive Care and a nearby druggist, Ron Mason, said he confronted the Purdue rep in early 2001 soon after his pharmacy had been robbed of OxyContin for the second time. During the first holdup, which occurred in 1999, a thief entered the store, put a gun to the head of a drugstore employee, and demanded OxyContin by name.

"I told him [Wilson], 'You know where this is going and that people are abusing this drug, but you are getting your commission on sales,'" recalled Mason in an interview with the *New York Times* in late 2001.

Wilson stopped speaking to him, Mason recounted. By June 2001, DEA officials, after a yearlong investigation, had gathered enough information to suspend the narcotics prescribing licenses of the doctors who worked at Comprehensive Care, effectively shutting down the pain clinic. Eight physicians employed there were subsequently indicted on criminal charges of illegally prescribing OxyContin and other controlled drugs.

Despite the agency's ongoing investigation of the clinic, the value of OxyContin prescriptions written in the Myrtle Beach area boomed. In fact, internal Purdue documents obtained by the *New York Times* showed that OxyContin sales in the Myrtle Beach area during the first three months of 2001 had grown by $1 million, a sum that was $300,000 higher than the growth in sales during that same period in any other company sales territory in the United States. As it turned out, right around the time that Ron Mason confronted Eric Wilson in his drugstore, Wilson was the top-ranked rep on Purdue's sales force. A Myrtle Beach physician would later say that Wilson told him that doctors working at Comprehensive Care accounted for about 40 percent of the OxyContin sales in his territory.

When asked in late 2001 by a *Times* reporter about Comprehensive Care and the large growth in OxyContin prescribing in Myrtle Beach, Purdue executives issued a statement that defended the company's action with respect to the clinic. The company also said that Mr. Wilson had been among those sales reps working in areas believed by the company to have a high potential for OxyContin abuse who had received added training in December 2000.

"Some have suggested that when suspicions are raised about a particular physician or practice, our sales representatives should stop calling on them," company officials said in the statement. "That certainly would have been better from a perception standpoint, but if a doctor is intent on prescribing our medication inappropriately, such activity would continue regardless of whether we contacted the doctor or not."

For his part, Eric Wilson, the sales rep, acknowledged in a statement released through Purdue in late 2001 that area druggists had expressed concerns to him about Comprehensive Care. Wilson said he had reported those concerns to his superiors but that it was decided that he should keep calling on its doctors because it was believed that "legitimate services were being provided to many patients in pain." He also told the *Times*, "If any of the doctors of this clinic have abused their prescribing privileges, then they have exploited all of us."

The subsequent trial of three doctors who had worked at Comprehensive Care raised questions about just how many legitimate pain patients were among its clientele. By then, five physicians associated with the facility, including Comprehensive Care's owner, Dr. David Michael Woodward, had already pleaded guilty to charges of illegally prescribing controlled drugs.

On the witness stand, Woodward, who had struck a plea bargain with prosecutors in exchange for his testimony, described Comprehensive Care as a thinly disguised dope-dealing enterprise where the customer was king.

"Did patients ever come in requesting particular prescriptions?" a prosecutor asked Woodward.

"Yes, sir, they did."

"What would they request?"

"The things that were requested the most were OxyContin, was the number one. And then second to that in terms of narcotics would be the Lorcet-type drugs, hydrocodones, by brand name. But the other popular things requested was Xanax, benzodiazepines like Valium, and Valium itself. So the top four would be OxyContin, Lorcet, Xanax, and Valium."

"How would you respond to the requests?"

"We tried to accommodate the patient," Woodward responded. "We were in the business essentially of selling prescriptions, and we wanted a patient to be happy."

There is no reason to believe that Woodward was so forthcoming in any talks he had with Eric Wilson. But that wasn't the point. Purdue's internal documents show that it didn't have a stated policy for many years that actively discouraged reps from calling on doctors under investigation for illegal prescribing.

Several former Purdue sales officials recalled that the drugmaker never forced them to visit a physician whom they suspected of improperly prescribing narcotics. Instead, those ex–sales officials said that the drugmaker left such decisions up to a rep's discretion. Such a laissez-faire approach, however, was fraught with conflict; a rep walking away from a physician was also walking away from income.

But in mid-2001, during the explosion of publicity about OxyContin pill mills, Purdue made some policy changes. The company told its sales force it might withhold commissions paid on OxyContin prescriptions written by doctors under investigation for inappropriately or illegally prescribing the painkiller. But by then two years had passed since the arrest of Dr. Frank Fisher and since the issue of sales rep commissions apparently was raised.

Purdue executives have never discussed what took place at that time, nor have they really said why they decided to institute the policy changes. One can only presume they had decided, as they had with their decision to drop OxyContin's labeling claim, that the "appropriate time" had arrived.

Just how far Purdue has put its new policies in the past is anyone's guess. Company executives wouldn't say when asked how much money they have docked or demanded back from the sales reps whose physicians were subsequently convicted of illegally prescribing. That accounting ledger, like the rest of Purdue's books, is apparently still private.

By 2003, Purdue executives were also struggling with another issue affecting all narcotics makers—should they add the opiate blocker naloxone or a similarly acting substance called naltrexone to OxyContin to reduce its abuse?

It was hardly the first time company officials had confronted the issue. Back in 1993, two years before OxyContin was approved by the FDA, a meeting took place at which Curtis Wright, the FDA medical examiner, suggested to a group of company officials that "we should consider a combination of OxyContin and naloxone," an internal Purdue memorandum stated. Another memo from the same year also makes reference to Wright's suggestion "for a combination (Oxycodone-Naltrexone) line extension product." Those suggestions apparently did not make much headway.

But by late 2001, Purdue executives were intensely reviewing the issue of adding an opiate blocker—much as Sterling Drug did with Talwin—to OxyContin. The decision was a complex one that raised significant economic, legal, and regulatory questions. And the problems involving OxyContin were even more complicated than those that had affected Talwin. While that drug was abused by hard-core addicts injecting it, OxyContin's misuse involved both recreational users and patients snorting the drug or chewing it.

The RADARS panel created by Purdue met in late 2001 to

discuss the issues surrounding the use of potential versions of OxyContin containing an opiate blocker, which had been code-named by the drugmaker "OXU," a copy of the group's report showed. The document also discusses another proposed product code-named "OpioidX," whose identity is not clear. Some of the issues raised in the RADARS panel report are as follows:

• Will the addition of opioid antagonists which indicates high abuse potential discourage some physicians from prescribing the product, and scare some patients away from using it?

• Even though the [existing OxyContin] label is very clear that crushing the tablets should be avoided there are bound to be elderly individuals who by accident do so. Those individuals will have a strong adverse event with the new combinations. What are the rates of accidental crushing of OxyContin?

• Once oxu and opioidX products become available, will the nonantagonist products [such as the existing version of OxyContin] remain on the market, providing a choice to physicians and patients? If both products are available, how much will the combination products reduce problems since 'script docs and doctor shoppers will demand the nonantagonist product?

• What is the effect of crushing the pellets that are used in the Palladone [timed-release] delivery system?

• What if any systems will be in place to study the effectiveness of the combination products in reducing misuse/abuse/dependence? How will RADARS be involved? Will RADARS have enough baseline data to be able to determine efficacy by the time the products are launched?

In its conclusions, the group reported:

> Despite the concerns expressed above, the RADARS [external advisory board] agrees that there could be considerable political and public health benefit if even a few individuals refrain from abusing the product or a few lives are saved by preventing an overdose. However, it must be remembered that theses [sic] products are not "waterproof" and at best are "water repellent." Overall, a risk benefit ratio must be established for the new products. It is essential to have a system in place to detect and respond to early evidence of abuse/dependence since no product is going to be effective against the determined addict.

Not long afterward, Purdue began holding focus groups with physicians, much as it did prior to marketing OxyContin, to get their feedback on their interests and concerns about prescribing a version of the drug with an opiate blocker. Physician reception was decidedly lukewarm, according to a memorandum describing those meetings. Several doctors said their need for such a drug was limited or questioned whether it would prove effective with patients who abuse OxyContin by chewing it.

There were also political and policy risks in marketing a modified form of OxyContin at the same time as the regular painkiller or in place of it. For example, one company document noted that the availability of both drugs not only might confuse doctors and reduce the number of prescriptions written, but might also have the effect of "erasing years of pain education efforts" as well as "increase awareness of abuse in patients" and end up "punishing patients." Meanwhile, the document raised the possibility that abuse of OXU could set off a "2nd Backlash Against OxyContin and Purdue" and potentially lead the FDA to pull both drugs off the market.

At the height of the OxyContin controversy, Purdue executives had announced with great fanfare that they were working furiously on a less-abusable form of OxyContin. But as Purdue executives likely knew by now, if they didn't before, nothing about the pain industry is that simple or that easy.

Preventing another disaster like OxyContin is not just the responsibility of drugmakers. Regulators and lawmakers have a part to play too.

By early 2003, for instance, FDA officials had started to keep a closer watch on the pain industry. The agency was set to formally adopt the recommendation from its advisory panel that a manufacturer of a new narcotic present it with a surveillance plan before marketing the drug so that any abuse, particularly by vulnerable groups such as young people, could be monitored.

One can only hope that the FDA won't repeat the same mistakes it made with OxyContin. Agency officials now insist that a manufacturer seeking to win a labeling claim suggesting that a narcotic offers a lower risk of abuse than equally powerful competitors will have to prove it by testing the drug on people before marketing the medication, not afterward, as was the case with OxyContin. In addition, the so-called approved medical uses of such drugs approved by the FDA—or their "indications," in agency parlance—might be more limited than those awarded OxyContin.

Only time will tell if regulators scrutinize such drugs more closely. But Purdue officials seemed to think they would. Indeed, company executives believed that from a competitive standpoint they had won an important commercial victory when they negotiated the changes to OxyContin's label with FDA officials in mid-2001, an internal company document shows.

"The action by the FDA to clarify the OxyContin Tablets labeling has created tremendous opportunities," a company budget-planning document declared. "In effect, the FDA has expanded the indication for OxyContin Tablets to any patient with moderate to severe, around-the-clock persistent pain, provided that the pain is moderate to severe and expected to be for an extended duration. This broad labeling is likely to never again be available for an opioid seeking FDA approval. This may give OxyContin a competitive advantage. This is a positive action which helps to combat the negative reports perpetuated by the media."

Meanwhile, the OxyContin episode revived legislative interest in prescription monitoring systems in several states including Virginia and Florida. Not surprisingly, some veterans of the pain management movement issued their customary jeremiads about the "chilling effect" such systems would produce.

But some of those who had previously questioned the value of monitoring, such as the University of Wisconsin's David Joranson, had by now climbed on the bandwagon. For them, the chill on narcotics prescribing created by the OxyContin episode was far more worrisome than reasonable efforts to catch bad doctors running pill mills or patients who "doctor-shopped" to collect multiple narcotics prescriptions. Purdue executives, to their credit, were a lone voice within the pharmaceutical industry lobbying on behalf of such programs.

It was hardly a coincidence that the states that experienced the worst outbreaks of OxyContin abuse—places like Florida, Kentucky, Maine, and Virginia—were those that didn't have a prescription monitoring system in place or were just setting one up when the drug's use exploded. But it would be overly simplistic to assume that regulators in states that had systems—New York and California, for instance—headed off OxyContin's misuse there because they were prompted by warning blips on their monitoring screens to take action.

Instead, prescription monitoring does appear to shape the psyches of doctors, as pain management advocates have claimed. But whether it causes a "chilling" effect or simply creates more cautious attitudes is another matter. One marketing firm told Purdue executives in 1995 that physicians from Texas, a state with monitoring, had said during focus groups that they were extremely unlikely to use OxyContin for noncancer pain. They said that not only didn't they want to be scrutinized by regulators, but they felt they could treat many pain conditions with medications less prone to abuse than a Schedule II narcotic. The real opportunities for OxyContin, the marketing group said, lay elsewhere, in states without monitoring where doctors already used Schedule II narcotics more liberally. One need only look to events in Maine, Virginia, Florida, and Kentucky that didn't have systems or had just started ones to see they were right. Cheri Crowley, the DEA investigator, who headed the inquiry into Comprehensive Care, said she believed that if South Carolina had a monitoring system or if Purdue had shared its IMS Health data with her office the pill mill could have been shut down six months earlier. As it was, her investigators had to sort through dusty prescription records at pharmacies throughout the state to pull those written by the pain clinic's doctor, grueling and mind-numbing work that seems senseless in the age of computers.

In the end, Purdue executives such as David Haddox, Michael Friedman, and Howard Udell may have been right after all about OxyContin, though not in any way they had imagined or intended. The painkiller, they have long insisted, really wasn't unique. In truth, it was tragically commonplace. OxyContin wasn't a novel way of fighting pain but simply a different way of administering the oldest of mankind's painkillers, the fruit of the opium poppy. And as a result, it may have been predestined to take its place in line behind morphine, Dilaudid, and every other narcotic that had originally promised strong painkilling power with a lower risk of abuse and addiction.

Purdue executives, along with their army of allies and paid apologists, have insisted that OxyContin was really just one part of the overall problem of prescription drug abuse. They've said that it was important to put the OxyContin problem into "perspective" to give it proper "balance." One can't argue with that. But then again, they were the ones who marketed and sold OxyContin for years as a different drug, one somehow safer than competing narcotics. Ever since, they have campaigned to downplay the scope of the OxyContin fiasco much in the way that narcotics activists trivialized the addictive potential of those drugs.

OxyContin ranks among the biggest prescription drug disasters to occur in recent decades, one whose legacy in terms of altered lives may be felt for decades to come. Purdue executives were certainly right about one thing: their drug was now very much a part of the problem of prescription drug abuse. OxyContin had been woven into that fabric as quickly and deeply as possible. In fact, it has left an indelible stain, one that neither time nor money will ever cleanse.

AFTERWORD

This book grew out of articles I wrote about OxyContin for the *New York Times*. The more I reported about this drug, the more it became clear to me that it could serve as a window into the important issues of pain management and prescription drug abuse.

My goal was simple: to examine how and why the problems involving OxyContin had happened from the perspective and experiences of those whose lives the drug had touched. That cast, who people the pages of this book, includes pain management experts and patients, regulators and drug agents, and prescription drug abusers and their parents and neighbors.

Naturally, another major part of the OxyContin story lay inside Purdue, in the perceptions of its executives toward the storm gathering around the drug and the reasoning and timing for their decisions. On several occasions I interviewed Purdue executives such as Michael Friedman and David Haddox for the *Times*. When work on this book began, in the spring of 2002, I wrote to them, to other executives at Purdue, and to members of the Sackler family to tell them about this project and seek their participation in it.

To a person, they refused to be interviewed. Company officials also declined to respond to specific questions I submitted to them in writing. Throughout the course of this project, the company's posture remained unchanged. I was disappointed by that decision because I would have welcomed their involvement. It has long been my belief, as well as my experience, that the input of all the actors in a story can only enrich it.

Nonetheless, I can't say I was surprised. Soon after I began reporting for the *Times* about OxyContin, Purdue executives began to complain about those articles to me, to my editors at the *Times*, and to others. Their basic charge was that they believed my reporting was inaccurate and unfair. They argued that my reporting also was unbalanced because it failed to give equal emphasis to the benefits that OxyContin was bringing to those suffering from chronic pain.

For example, in a letter to me dated January 9, 2003, Howard Udell wrote that he and other Purdue officials believed that an article I had written for the *Times* had failed to accurately report what I had been told, and that I had also "excerpted and slanted our words to support your clearly preconceived views." Mr. Udell wrote, "Those experiences play an important part in my decision and the decisions of my colleagues (on whose behalf I am responding) not to be interviewed by you again."

Companies, like individuals, have the right to choose the forums in which to publicly present their views, and Purdue is no different. I have no doubt that Purdue executives were unhappy with my reporting. But I also believe that it was critical to understand the company's role as well as its responsibilities, if any, for the OxyContin fiasco; this is simply what reporters are supposed to do.

In this book, I have sought to give a description of Purdue's efforts to reduce prescription drug abuse. However, the reader may wish to read about those programs in the company's own words. That material is available on Purdue's Web site, www.purduepharma.com.

It is my hope that the full story of what occurred inside Purdue will be known some day, captured not only in public pronouncements of corporate executives but also in disclosed internal documents. Such clarity is critical in assessing the performance of company officials. It might also help to serve as a guide that could prevent similar drug disasters in the future.

New York City
July 2003

SOURCES AND NOTES

This book was based on more than two hundred interviews and a review of thousands of pages of documents including court records, internal Purdue documents, scientific reports, journal articles, and both newspaper and magazine articles. Some of the material presented was originally reported or gathered for the *New York Times*, though the vast majority was gathered specifically for this book.

In reconstructing scenes where I was not present, I sought to interview numerous parties to an event or both participants in a conversation. That wasn't always possible, so I can't attest to the accuracy of each quoted word, but I have given the reader the source of these quotes.

Prologue: The Book of the Dead

The prologue is drawn from interviews with Dr. Fredric Hellman, the medical examiner for Delaware County, PA; Dr. William Massello, a medical examiner for the state of Virginia; and Linda Sullivan, the manager of toxicology at the Wuesthoff Reference Laboratories in Melbourne, FL. Ms. Sullivan was also profiled by Mary McLaclin in the *Palm Beach Post,* August 26, 2001.

Chapter One: Pill Hill

Much of this chapter is drawn from interviews with Lindsay Myers, Jane Myers, Sister Beth Davies, Sister Elizabeth Vines, Art Van Zee, Sue Ella Kobak, Larry Lavender, Vince Stravino, and Greg Stewart.

by April the figure had risen to 90 percent . . . Dennis Lee, Virginia Commonwealth attorney for Tazewell County, provided that estimate. Lee also said that forged $40 checks were so common that police officials joked, "We know where that $40 went."

315

the company filed a required report ...   Stravino's call to Purdue appears in an adverse drug reaction report filed by Purdue Pharma with the Food and Drug Administration. It notes that he made his initial call to the company on April 7, 2002.

he picked up a copy of the Boston Globe ...   Stravino read about OxyContin abuse in Washington County, Maine, in an article by Donna Gold in the *Globe* on May 21, 2000.

Chapter Two: Senior Night

Van Zee had learned from newspaper accounts ... Newspapers that published articles in the spring and summer of 2000 about OxyContin abuse included the *Portland Press Herald,* the *Roanoke Times,* the *Columbus Dispatch,* and the *Anchorage Daily News.*

"This probably will be your new Vicodin" ...   This quote from a law enforcement official appeared in an article by Steve Cannizaro that appeared in the *Times-Picayune* on June 27, 2000.

That August, Van Zee decided to write ...   Art Van Zee provided me with copies of his correspondence to Dr. J. David Haddox and Dr. Daniel Spyker. Van Zee recalled that he might have met Spyker when the physician was working at the Blue Ridge Poison Control Center.

Gate City scored first ...   The brief description of the game between Lee High and Gate City was taken from the *Powell Valley News,* a weekly newspaper in Pennington Gap.

In a cover letter, a physician named Susan Bertrand ...   Letter dated August 8, 2000.

"Among the remedies which it has pleased" ...   Susan Bertrand's quotation from Thomas Sydenham, while accurate in spirit, may not have have reflected a precise rendering of his words. In his exhaustive survey *Opium: A History* (St. Martin's Press, 1996), Martin Booth quoted Sydenham: "God, the giver of all good things, who hath granted to the human race, as a comfort in their afflictions, no medicine of the value of opium either in regard to the number of diseases it can control, or its efficiency in extirpating them ..."

David Haddox, the Purdue executive ...   Like other company executives, David Haddox declined to be interviewed for this book. He also declined to provide a list of people familiar with his career. Several of them, however, agreed to be interviewed.

pseudoaddiction ...   The term was first used by Haddox and his coauthor, Dr. David E. Weissman, in a paper titled "Opioid pseudoaddiction ... an iatrogenic syndrome," *Pain*, 1989.

a reporter at a small newspaper in southwestern Virginia ...   Theresa M. Clemons was the reporter at the *Richlands News-Press* who was contacted by David Haddox. Her first article about the explosion of OxyContin abuse in Tazewell County appeared in the *News-Press* on May 31, 2000. Haddox's quote regarding opioid addiction risks as being "one half of one percent" is from a follow-up article by Clemons that appeared on June 21, 2000.

The idea for the group had come from Susan Bertrand ...   Dr. Bertrand described the background of the Appalachian Pain Foundation during an interview I did with her in connection with an article about OxyContin for the *New York Times.*

The company was aware that several doctors ... were already under criminal investigation ...   Mary Baluss, a pain management advocate and lawyer in Washington, D.C., told me that several Purdue reps in Appalachia contacted her in mid-2000 and asked her to speak with physicians facing scrutiny over their prescribing. Baluss attended the Appalachian Pain Foundation's meeting in Richlands at the invitation of David Haddox, and on the way there she said they stopped off to see one of those physicians, Dr. Franklin Sutherland Jr. Not long afterward, Sutherland was indicted and convicted of illegally prescribing several drugs including OxyContin.

"We have never seen anything like this before" . . .   Dennis Lee's quote is taken from an article by Tom Angleberger in the *Roanoke Times,* September 25, 2000.

Chapter Three: A War against Pain

Many of the events depicted in this chapter are based on interviews with Dr. Russell K. Portenoy, who is the chief of pain and palliative care department at Mt. Sinai Medical Center in New York City. Anthony Guaimano and his wife, Joan, were kind enough to describe his battle with cluster headaches to me.

Pain is frequently described . . .   I have attempted only a brief and superficial accounting of the history of pain management and the medical science surrounding it. Along with Martin Booth's *Opium,* books that may be of interest to the general reader are *Why We Hurt; The Natural History of Pain* by Dr. Frank T. Vertosick Jr. and *The Culture of Pain* by David B. Morris.

80 percent of those people . . .   The statistics on the unreliability of X rays in the detection of back pain were cited by Dennis Turk in his paper "Clinicians' Attitudes about Prolonged Use of Opioids and the Issue of Patient Heterogeneity" in the *Journal of Pain and Symptom Management,* 1996

350 researchers from around the world . . .   It was Dr. John Bonica, one of the founders of modern pain management, who put together the 1973 meeting near Seattle that led to the formation a year later of the International Association for the Study of Pain. My very quick rendering of pain thought through the years is drawn from Bonica's *Management of Pain,* a textbook considered a bible for the field.

doctors believed that opium was benign . . .   The descriptions of paregoric, laudanum, and Thomas Sydenham's laudanum recipe are all drawn from Martin Booth's *Opium.*

soldier's disease . . .   Civil War veterans were only one of the groups that included significant numbers of opiate addicts. According to historians like David Musto, white, middle-class women represented another major one. Musto's book *The American Disease* (Yale University Press, 1973) is regarded as the classic text on the impact over the years of government laws and regulations like the Harrison Act of 1914 on narcotics use, their abuse, and physician behavior.

Dr. Saunders opened the first facility . . . in the final months of life . . .   Dr. Cicely Saunders was a remarkable woman. A nurse who cared for the dying in sterile hospital environments, she decided to go back to medical school to get a degree so that doctors would be forced to pay attention to her ideas. The first hospice in the United States opened in 1981 near New Haven, Connecticut.

most notably Memorial Sloan-Kettering . . .   While better cancer pain care started in England, the cancer pain researchers at Memorial Sloan-Kettering prided themselves on taking a far more scientific approach than their British colleagues. They constantly ran tests on patients to determine which substances worked best. In the early 1980s, for example, Memorial Sloan-Kettering was one of two hospitals that experimentally gave heroin to cancer patients while Congress debated whether to legalize its medical use. As it turned out, heroin, which is derived from morphine and breaks back down into it shortly after entering the body, wasn't any more effective.

"chronic pain in litigation" . . .   The description of the rapidly rising rate of back pain during the 1990s was cited in an article by Elizabeth Rosenthal in the *New York Times,* December 29, 1992. That same article also cited research by Dr. Michael Weintraub that had appeared in the *American Journal of Pain Management,* which looked at pain complaints by plaintiffs in lawsuits. It was Dr. Weintraub who said that patients may get subconsciously attached to pain

because of the prospect of financial rewards and suggested that "chronic pain in litigation" be viewed as a distinct syndrome.

multidisciplinary approach . . . Descriptions of this approach were provided by Dr. Hubert L. Rosomoff, director of the Comprehensive Pain and Rehabilitation Center in Miami; Dennis Turk; and Barry Cole.

"opiophobia" . . . The apparent origin of the term *opiophobia* is an article written by Dr. John P. Morgan in a 1986 issue of the journal *Controversies in Alcoholism and Substance Abuse*. Dr. Morgan's article was entitled "American Opiophobia: Customary Underutilization of Opioid Analgesics."

handing him a Bronx telephone book . . . Russell Portenoy's 1986 study of drugstores was entitled "Unavailability of Narcotic Analgesics for Ambulatory Patients in New York City."

Foley . . . a seminal figure . . . Dr. Kathleen M. Foley, along with her contributions to the field of cancer pain treatment, became a seminal figure in advocacy efforts to improve the care of the terminally ill, a field known as palliative care. She declined to be interviewed for this book. Her observations and comments cited in this chapter are drawn from a 1996 oral history she gave for the John C. Liebeskind History of Pain Collection at UCLA. She was interviewed by Marcia L. Meldrum.

A report he published in 1986 . . . The study by Portenoy and Foley appeared in *Pain*.

the holy scientific trinity . . . The three studies cited by Portenoy, pain management activists, Purdue Pharma, and other drug companies in support of extremely minimal risk of iatrogenic addiction are "Drug Dependency in Patients with Chronic Headache," which appeared in *Headache* 17 (1977), 12–14; "Addiction Rare in Patients Treated with Narcotics," a letter in the *New England Journal of Medicine* 302 (1980), 123; and "Management of Pain during Debridement; A Survey of U.S. Burn Units" in *Pain* 13 (1982), 267–80.

In a series of influential papers . . . David Joranson's writing on the issue of prescription monitoring systems has appeared in a number of publications, including the *American Pain Society Bulletin* and the *Journal of Pharmaceutical Care in Pain and Symptom Control*. He declined to be interviewed for this book.

Purdue contributed half a million . . . This contribution to the joint committee of the American Pain Society and the American Academy of Pain Management is found in a Purdue budget document.

Another recipient of industry funds . . . was David Joranson . . . This information is drawn from documents obtained from the University of Wisconsin under that state's open records law. They also show that Joranson served as a paid consultant to several narcotics manufacturers, principally Purdue.

Chapter Four: Magic Bullets

Much of the information about the background of the narcotics industry and the development of high thebaine–yielding poppies in Tasmania was drawn from interviews with Gene Haslip, Dr. Marshall Smalley, Lloyd Nystrom, Raymond Stratmeyer, and Herbert Schaepe.

blamed Percodan misuse . . . for up to one-quarter of all drug addiction in California . . . Gladwin Hill, *New York Times*, June 2, 1963. At the time, the problem of Percodan abuse was blamed by many observers on the drug's overaggressive promotion by its manufacturer and a change in California rules that made it easier to prescribe the drug.

FDA examiner Curtis Wright . . .   At the time of this writing, Mr. Wright was working for Purdue Pharma.

the FDA didn't require narcotics makers to run abuse studies . . .   In the case of OxyContin, the agency, which was concerned about addicts injecting OxyContin, did require Purdue to run tests to determine whether talc was precipitated when the drug was dissolved. It was.

Purdue had not done so for MS Contin . . .   In a letter to Howard Udell, I asked why Purdue had sought the reduced abuse liability claim for OxyContin but not MS Contin. He didn't respond.

The Farm . . .   The history of the federal effort to develop a nonaddicting painkiller and the establishment of prison-hospitals for addicts is a fascinating byroad in the history of drug abuse prevention. For more, see *Creating the American Junkie* by Caroline Jean Acker (Johns Hopkins University Press, 2002).

The company said its findings were based on testing . . . Talwin . . .   Sterling Drug's premarket testing of Talwin is described by Jane Brody in the *New York Times*, June 27, 1967.

to convince cancer specialists to switch from MS Contin to OxyContin . . .   Purdue's initial marketing study for OxyContin is laid out in a 1995 company document called the OxyContin Launch Plan.

one company marketing document from 1996 . . .   Each year, Purdue produced a document that laid out its marketing goals and strategies for the year ahead, including a budget for programs it planned to underwrite.

Partners Against Pain . . .   This patient-outreach program was created by Purdue in 1995.

two thousand to three thousand doctors would attend those meetings . . .   Dr. Howard Heit provided that estimate to me when I interviewed him in 2001 for the *New York Times*.

"1 percent or less" . . .   This figure is repeatedly cited in internal Purdue material.

"If I Only Had a Brain" . . .   Jim Lang's memo is dated November 4, 1996.

70 percent of our theft crimes . . .   Sheriff Gary Parson's letter is dated November 13, 2000.

Chapter Five: Chicken and Biscuits

a sheet of paper that he handed to Haddox . . .   The list of suggestions that Art Van Zee gave to David Haddox was dated November 20, 2000.

the tiny town of St. Paul . . .   The meeting attended by the Yale professors, David Fiellin and Richard Schottenfeld, was held on November 30, 2000, at the Oxbow Center in St. Paul.

This one wasn't going to Purdue . . .   Art Van Zee's letter to Deborah Leiderman, the FDA official, was dated December 3, 2000.

Chapter Six: Hot Spots

Sister Beth started the meeting . . .   The account of the town meeting at Lee High is drawn from an article that appeared in the *Powell Valley News*.

a lengthy, front-page article in the New York Times *. . .*   That article appeared on March 5, 2001. It was written by Melody Petersen and me.

"We were getting creamed" . . .   Robin Hogen, Purdue's spokesman, made those comments during a 2002 conference held by Bulldog Reporter, an oddly named public relations group. His speech

was entitled "How to Respond When Your Product Comes Under Attack: OxyContin Fights Back."

in publications including the New York Times . . .   A team of Purdue executives visited the *Times* in mid-2001 to complain about the paper's handling of the OxyContin story. Along with my stories, the company was particularly incensed by an article by my colleague Paul Tough that appeared in the *Times Sunday Magazine* on July 29, 2001. At the meeting, the paper's editors said they believed that the coverage had been fair.

"a new standard in corporate responsibility" . . .   The comments of Purdue officials to the *Hart-ford Courant* were reported in *American Health Line*, July 19, 2001.

Van Zee had brought another man to the meeting . . .   This man agreed to be interviewed on the condition that he not be identified.

"I want to show you this" . . .   Sister Beth Davies kept a copy of the ad prepared by Purdue.

Chapter Seven: Kiddie Dope

Michael Friedman wrote to Nagel . . .   His first letter to Laura Nagel was dated March 8, 2001.

"As we discussed at the meeting" . . .   Friedman's letter following up on Purdue's first meeting with Nagel was dated April 2, 2001.

overdose deaths in Florida from prescription narcotics . . .   The data on Florida drug deaths was reported by Doris Bloodsworth in the *Orlando Sentinel*, May 27, 2001.

Thomas Constantine . . .   The unhappiness of DEA agents with Mr. Constantine was reported by Gordon Wilkin in *U.S. News & World Report*, June 5, 1995.

DEA announced a . . . sweeping program . . .   See my article in the *New York Times*, May 1, 2001.

Woodworth was squaring off against David Haddox . . .   Terry Woodworth and David Haddox debated each other on the *CBS Early Show*, May 3, 2001.

"USA Today is planning an editorial" . . .   Howard Udell's note to Laura Nagel was dated June 11, 2001; the paper's editorial appeared on June 13, 2001.

Joranson's study . . .   David Joranson's study appeared in *JAMA* on April 5, 2000.

Chapter Eight: A Tacit Understanding

"Are you a real doctor?" . . .   This response to Art Van Zee's recall petition was reported by Laurence Hammack in the *Roanoke Times*, November 25, 2001.

Jick would say years later . . .   Dr. Jick made those comments when I interviewed him.

Dr. Richard G Paolino . . .   For more about the Paolino case, see Alicia A. Caldwell, Mark Bowden, and Elisa Ung in the *Philadelphia Inquirer*, July 29, 30, and 31, 2001.

The Bensalem hearing . . .   This hearing was held on August 28, 2001. I didn't attend, but my descriptions of Michael Friedman's demeanor and facial expression are drawn from a videotape of the hearing.

Foley had seen a television documentary . . .   On December 12, the CBS newsmagazine *48 Hours* aired a documentary entitled "Addicted." The following day, MTV aired a related OxyContin documentary entitled "True Life: I'm Hooked on OxyContin." It was not clear which one she saw.

Schnoll said he had "no idea" . . . Both Schnoll and Nathaniel Paul Katz spoke at the 2002 conference of th e American Society of Addiction Medicine. I attended it as a guest of the Wake Forest University Addiction Studies Program for Journalists.

Chapter Nine: The Secrets of Dendur

Dr. Arthur M. Sackler testified . . . Sackler testified January 30, 1962, before the subcommittee on antitrust and monopoly of the Senate Committee on the Judiciary.

the company's sole shareholder was Else Sackler . . . Medical & Science Communications Associates Inc. was originally known as Communications Associates. It changed its name on September 16, 1955, and it is that document that identifies Else Sackler's role. A similarly named entity that would operate as a holding company until Arthur Sackler's death was Medical and Science Communications Development Corporation. A 1968 stock certificate shows that its stock was held in trust by Else Sackler, Mortimer Sackler, and Raymond Sackler for the benefit of Carol Sackler, Arthur and Else's first child.

Creedmoor State Hospital . . . For more on the research work of Arthur, Mortimer, and Raymond Sackler, see the *New York Times*, November 2, 1951; September 8, 1957; and April 15, 1976.

multipage color insert in JAMA . . . Arthur Sackler was one of the original inductees in the Medical Advertising Hall of Fame. Some of his achievements are described in one of the group's publications, *Medicine Ave*. William G. Castagnoli was kind enough to provide a copy.

The American Connection . . . John Pekkanen's excellent book is a study of legislative battling and pharmaceutical industry lobbying that shaped the Controlled Substances Act.

he received bonus payments . . . Librium and Valium . . . Michael Sonnenreich, Arthur Sackler's lawyer, told me this during an interview. I mentioned to him that I had heard that Sackler received a royalty based on each pill sold; he said that wasn't the case but acknowledged incentive bonuses were paid when sales reached certain benchmarks.

"happy baby vitamin" . . . The documents related to this bizarre episode are contained within the hearing record of the Kefauver committee.

Medical Tribune . . . For a quick flavor of the newspaper's slant, see Morton Mintz, *Washington Post,* March 31, 1968.

"Schizophrenics 'Wild'" . . . See Tamar Levin, *New York Times*, July 27, 1987.

The FDA investigated . . . The comments about the article are drawn from a presentation by James C. Morrison, deputy director, Office of Drug Standards, on June 18, 1986.

Mortimer and Raymond were fired . . . See the *New York Times*, May 8, 1953.

"When Spring Comes" . . . I found this advertising card on the Internet.

Glutavite Corporation . . . The company's original name was Medical Promotion Productions.

John Lear . . . His classic articles in the *Saturday Review* about the pharmaceutical industry should be required reading in every journalism and civics class. One benefit of working on this book was discovering them. For his reports about the pharmaceutical industry or the Sacklers, see the *Saturday Review*, January 3, 1959; February 7, 1959; June 4, 1960; July 2, 1960; March 3, 1962; and October 6, 1962.

To avoid paying United States taxes . . . Gertraud Sackler's claim was contained in a court filing in New York State Supreme Court.

The ownership of MD Publications . . .   The precise transactions involving the ownership interests in MD Publications are not clear, but estate records indicate that a significant stake in the
company was apparently held at one point by Mortimer and Raymond Sackler or entities that
they controlled. That interest was transferred back into Arthur Sackler's estate after his death
as part of a larger swap and sale of Sackler family–owned assets.

Chapter Ten: The Body Count

"We don't believe there is a cause for panic" . . .   That comment by an FDA official was reported
in a story I did for the *New York Times*, April 15, 2002.

Robin Hogen . . . could barely contain himself . . .   Hogen's comments about the soon-to-be-
announced hiring of Rudolph Giuliani was made to the public relations group Bulldog Reporter.

Rudolph Giuliani . . .   He declined through a spokesperson to be interviewed for this book.

"The mayor and I just met with Asa Hutchinson" . . .   Bernard Kerik's comments were reported
by Chris Smith in *New York magazine*, September 15, 2002.

True copies of all communications . . .   Several reporters including myself petitioned to receive the
file of Bob Butterworth's investigation into Purdue under Florida's open records law. Purdue
sought to block the release of those records but lost in court. The file contained, among other
documents, the company's marketing budget plans for the years 1996 to 2002; notes from the
interview with William Gergely, a former Purdue rep; and the letters between Jody Collins and
Jon Sale.

Chapter Eleven: Purple Peelers

"Too much heroin and too many Oxycontins" . . .   The article quoting William Beatty was written
by Linda Harris and appeared in the *Weirton Daily Times* on April 20,1999.

Scientists from the University of British Columbia had uncovered the problem . . .   The report documenting the abuse of MS Contin was conducted by Dr. Amin Sajan, Dr. Trevor Corneil, and
Dr. Stefan Gryzbowski from the school's Department of Family Practice.

Frank Fisher's hearing . . .   Those hearings stretched over a four-month period in the spring of
1999.

the bulletin written by Ron Portash . . .   Mr. Portash sent out his warning to doctors in Cambria
County, PA, about the growing abuse of OxyContin on August 5, 1999. In a later note to me,
he said that he had included information in it about Ultram and Dilaudid so as "not to focus
solely on OxyContin, and at that time risk a lawsuit from the pharmaceutical industry."

Leon Dulion first called on Graves . . .   Dulion was deposed on October 9, 2001, prior to the trial
of Dr. James F. Graves. His deposition testimony was far more sweeping and colorful that his
later testimony at Graves' trial.

"you've done a good job of remaining 'Audible Ready'" . . .   Mark Radcliffe, a district manager,
offered that compliment to a Purdue sales rep in Tennessee, Brian Purdue, when assessing his
sales techniques during visits to doctors and pharmacists in late August 2000.

The South Florida Sun-Sentinel *reported that its review of medical examiner data* . . .   The newspaper's findings were contained in a series of enterprising stories reported by Nancy McVicar
and Fred Schulte that appeared on May 12, 13, and 14, 2002.

Chapter Twelve: New Beginnings

a "misunderstanding" . . .   In mid-2003, well after reviewing the warning letter from the FDA, Purdue ran a two-page correction in the *Journal of the American Medical Association* that addressed its problem ads.

Chapter Thirteen: The Pain Industry

British regulators handed down . . .   The antitrust ruling against Napp Pharmaceuticals was issued on March 30, 2001. It was upheld on January 15, 2002, though the fine was reduced.

The drug involved was Ultram . . .   The program developed by Ortho-McNeil to monitor the abuse of Ultram is described in a paper prepared by the company's consultants that appeared in *Drug and Alcohol Dependence* 57 (1999), 7–22.

a pain clinic in Myrtle Beach . . .   Events at Comprehensive Care and Pain Management, as well as the growing sales of OxyContin in Myrtle Beach, were the subject of an article I reported for the *New York Times* that appeared on December 10, 2001.